This book is dedicated to my parents
Anne and Jimmy Rooney.

Table of Contents

Acknowledgements: i
Warning-Disclaimer ii
Preface iii
Introduction 1
1. Exploring your core foundations. How healthy are yours? 9
2. Nutritional Healing; The basics. 15
3. Specific foods to heal the foundation 33
4. Supplements to support the foundation 47
5. Stretches for the foundation 57
6. Corrective Exercises 77
7. Stress: Dealing with the "fight/ flight or freeze "response 105
8. Mindfulness with Movement 119
9. Family systems and tribal/Ancestral contracts 131
10. Mindfulness about your Behaviour 147
11. Archetypes of the foundation 171
12. Health conditions and Diseases of the foundation 187
13. Final thoughts 225
References 243
About the Author: Clare Rooney 255

Go to my Website www.ClareRooney.com and sign up for a free report on fat loss.

© Clare Rooney 2015. All Rights reserved.

Acknowledgements:

I want to thank the people who have been amazing contributors to my journey in the field of health, wellness and training.

I wish to thank Charles Poliquin who I interned with over a period of 10 years. The vast wealth of knowledge I learned from him was literally priceless.

I wish to thank Paul Chek who taught me the true meaning of holistic health. His approach to assessing clients for exercise purposes has been indispensable to me in my personal training practice.

I wish to thank Bill Wolcott, the founder of Metabolic Typing who taught me the value and necessity for individualized nutrition.

I wish to thank Brent Anderson of Polestar Education whereby I have learned the true power of mindful movement.

I wish to thank all of the clients I have worked with over the years. I have learned the most valuable lessons from them.

Most importantly I wish to thank my parents for instilling in me the value of education and for their unrelenting support through all of my life.

Warning-Disclaimer

The information is this book is for educational purposes only. Consult your medical doctor before considering any of the nutritional or supplemental nutrients suggested. Not all exercises are suitable for everyone. Consult your exercise physiologist or physiotherapist to assess suitability to do the exercises, especially if you are already injured or new to exercise. The information contained in this book is not a substitute for medical advice.

Preface

A code is defined as:

"A systematically arranged and comprehensive collection of laws."

Source : http://www.thefreedictionary.com

In the modern world health is a destination that only a lucky few can ever hope to arrive at. A Shangri-La for the wealthy individuals and Hollywood stars who have specialist doctors, personal chefs and wellness gurus on speed dial.

Why is it that even though we are living in the information age with countless gigabytes of information at our finger tips that we as human beings have never been sicker, fatter or more medicated than any other era in history?

The problem, my dear friends, is not a lack of information but the ability to apply that information in the perfect sequence, correct amount and optimal time that will crack our personal health conundrum. Working on food allergies without addressing the fight/flight or freeze response is for example a waste of time. One simply develops a new set of allergies and results are temporary at best.

Trying to be mindful while not being anchored in your body is like looking through a pair of binoculars without focusing the lens. When you are not in your body your awareness is a distorted lens, no matter how present you try to be. So what's the solution? We now know that that which affects the body affects the mind and vice versa. This is one of the reasons that mindfulness classes have become so popular. What is not so widely known is that the feedback loop between body and mind is up to 90/10 in the direction of body to brain[1]. The emerging field of neurogastroenterology is directing our attention to the fact that our brains may well be a very misplaced focus and that a happy body may be the true route to a happy mind. So if you can bring that body to what it truly desires, a sense of safety, mindfulness arises spontaneously without any effort.

"Cracking the mind/body code" puts you firmly on the right road to health and happiness. Instead of dropping you randomly by parachute into a jungle of information, you are shown step by step the exercises, nutritional practices, and awareness's that will become the bed rock on which you build ever evolving levels of health and wellness.

Introduction

Who this book is for

You are a Physical, Mental, Emotional and Spiritual Being. To achieve the greatest levels of health and wellness we need to not only focus on our physical body but on other aspects of our being. What is required is a balancing of the seemingly dualistic western & eastern traditions.

As a student of western empirical science and a curious explorer of oriental mysticism it has always been my natural tendency to see the connections and similarities between these two apparently opposing views of the world. Many westerners or those who believe that only science can answer the most interesting questions about life, health and the meaning of existence have dismissed any alternative perspective even if that perspective is talking about the same thing (albeit with a different metaphor or use of symbolism).

This book is for those who have an open mind, appreciate good science and are willing to learn from other cultures and viewpoints. Call it a holistic approach if you will. If you're a diehard scientist who refuses to see the world from any other vista, this book might offer some insights into how some eastern practices can be explained in light of current scientific evidence…..

I have drawn on knowledge from both Eastern and Western traditions, to give an alternate but complimentary view of how the body works optimally to manifest higher levels of health and wellness. Consider this a manual for doing and living! I encourage you to try the exercises, even if you think they don't apply to you.

"Sooner or later you're going to realize just as I did that there's a difference between knowing the path and walking the path."

Morpheus

I am going to use the Chakra system, as used in Ayurvedic and Yogic traditions for millennia, as the basic template to work with. I'll weave into it the science of how to heal the body using movement, nutrition, herbs and other techniques that will complement each other.

"Not everything that can be counted counts and not everything that counts can be counted."

Albert Einstein

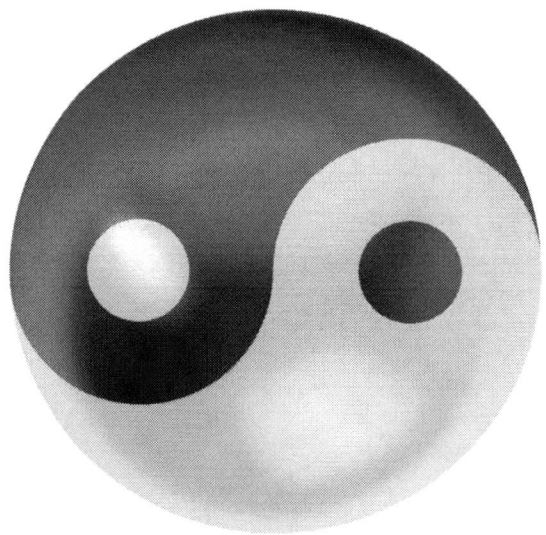

Figure 1: Source: FOTOLIA

The Yin Yang symbol from the East depicting the polar nature of the Universe

The Atomic structure below shows the Western idea of Polarity with positively charged protons and negatively charged electrons in Atoms.

Atom structure

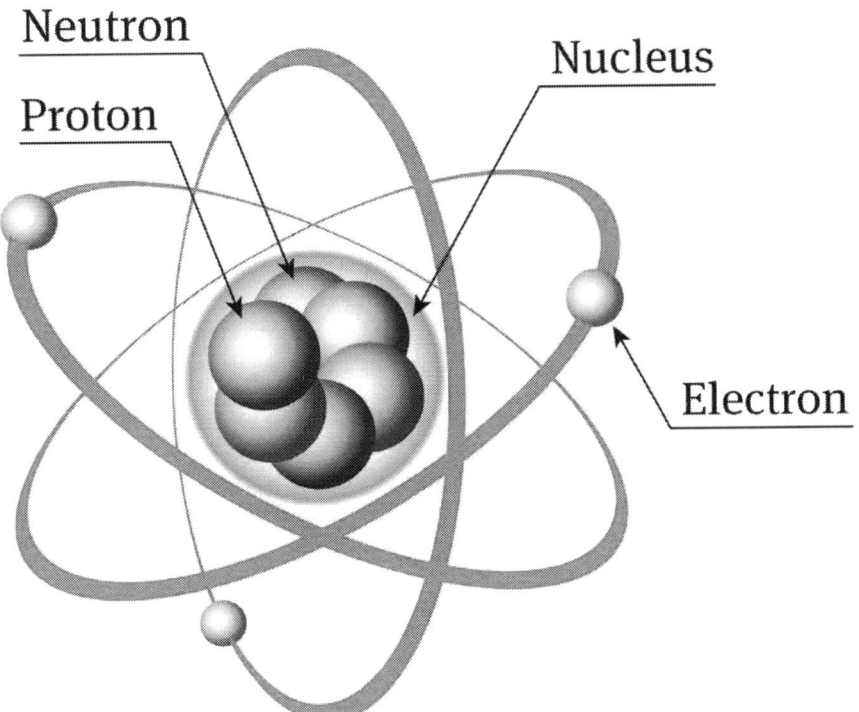

Figure 2: Source: FOTOLIA

Everything is Energy

"If you want to find the secrets of the Universe, think in terms of energy, frequency and vibration."
Nikola Tesla

It has been said that all of science is about condensing multiple principles and laws into a singular unifying principle -that great mathematical equation that explains everything. One of the most powerful equations to come out of the 20th Century is Albert Einstein's theory of Relativity; $E = MC^2$

It means that energy is mass x the speed of light squared. So if we are going to have a decent understanding of the universe, we need to look at three things:

Energy (the capacity to do work)

Mass (the quantity of matter)

Light (the electromagnetic energy of many different wavelengths including the visible spectrum).

In training parameters we think of mass in terms of weight lifted in the gym. We fuel our bodies with energy-giving foods to ensure high levels of energy for training. Interestingly we tend not to think about the light part of the equation so much. That's beginning to change as we learn more about vitamin D, the benefits of light when we go for our infra-red sauna, or go out in the sunshine.

It turns out the whole of the chakra system is based on light! And the foundation stone of understanding of energy in Physics is the electromagnetic spectrum (of which the visible spectrum is part).

ELECTROMAGNETIC SPECTRUM

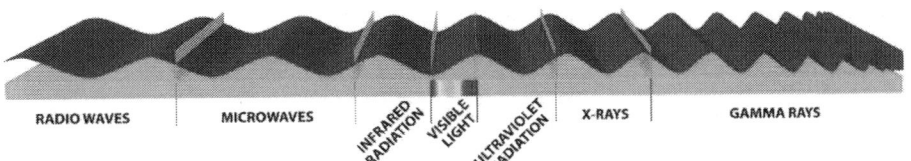

Figure 3: Source: FOTOLIA

What are Chakras?

The chakras of the human body are described as being energy vortexes or wheels that emanate from the body at different junctures.

The basic models of the chakra system depict 7 chakras. Some other systems show more, including minor chakras. I will use the basic 7 chakra model. The 7 chakras from bottom to top are Root or Base chakra, Sacral chakra, Solar Plexus, Heart chakra, Throat chakra, Third eye chakra and Crown chakra. The chakras are also associated with colours, just like the rainbow or when white light is passed through a prism.

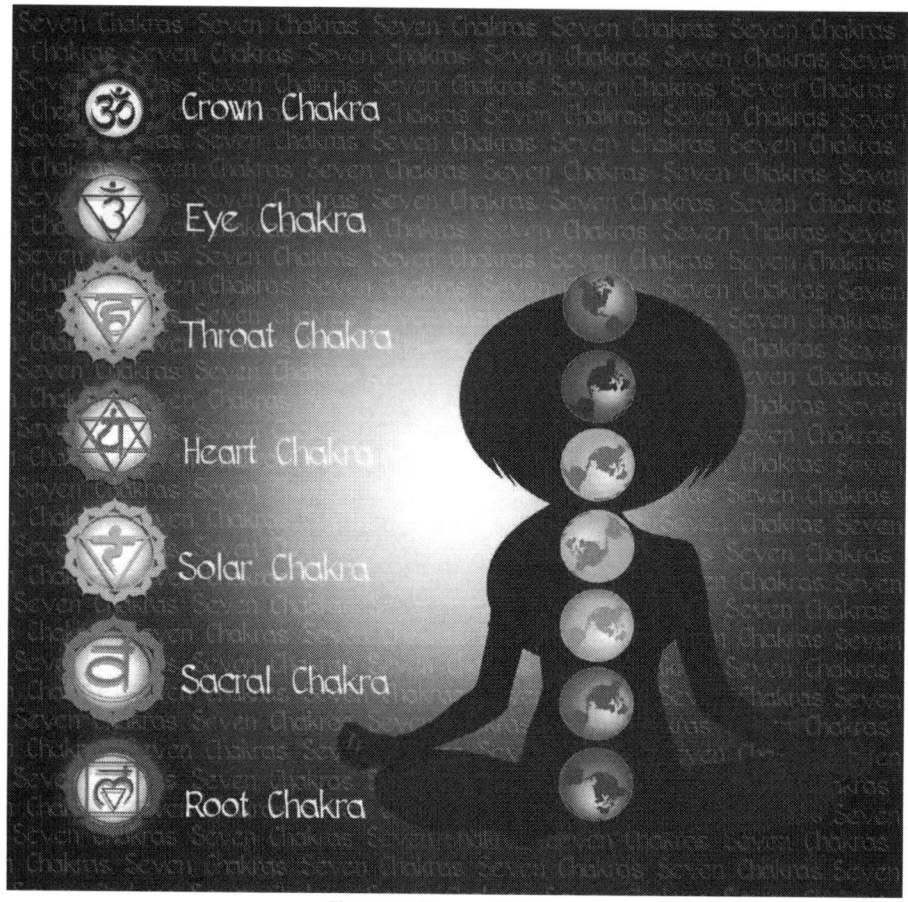

Figure 4: Source; FOTOLIA

Root or Base chakra is Red

Sacral Chakra is Orange

Solar Plexus is yellow

Heart Chakra is Green (sometimes also associated with Pink)

Throat chakra is sky Blue

Third eye is a deep indigo blue

Crown Chakra is Purple

From the electromagnetic spectrum we know that white light is comprised of several colours and each of these colours has its own frequency or unique energy fingerprint. The same can be said with the chakras. Each chakra or energy centre has unique energetic properties and resonates at a specific frequency.

The chakras correspond to different regions of the body. They are associated with different endocrine organs, nerve plexuses (bundles of nerves), mental and emotional states and even overall themes in life and behaviours.

If you wish to look into the science of the bodies energy field more deeply I suggest you look at the work of Dr Valerie Hunt PhD who has been studying the human aura (the field of electromagnetic energy emanating from and surrounding the human body) for several decades now. She has even developed sensitive instruments to measure it. Her conclusion after years of research is that all illness starts with a disturbance in the body's electromagnetic field:

"You're not going to have health if you don't have health in the electromagnetic field because this is the source. Biochemistry never gives you source."
Dr Valerie Hunt PhD

This book will focus on the root chakra and explore many of the methods that can be used in a complimentary way to optimise and heal this chakra. The more tools you implement, the faster your rate of progress will be, and the more enriching the process of transformation will be.

In working with the body's energy field (bio electromagnetic field), you get to the source of disturbances that lead to illness. So if a chakra is blocked, under-functioning or over active, disease is soon to follow.

The chakras are simply regions of this electromagnetic field that have a specific frequency of energy.

Chapter 1

Exploring your core foundations. How healthy are yours?

Every chakra influences us on all levels; mental, physical, emotional and spiritual. The root chakra encompasses what I call your core foundations. The key issues from which we create and generate our lives. The root chakras most obvious influence is on the physical (although it does have effects on the other 3 areas also). The root chakra is connected with all of the following:

Physical condition and health

Vitality

Strength

Body composition, lean mass versus fat mass

Health and functioning of the muscles and bones

Biomechanical issues such as flexibility, and stability.

Athletic ability

Ability to generate power (in the physical sense)

Ability to find/ generate food and shelter

All issues pertaining to safety

Physical reflexes

Fight/ flight or Freeze response

Financial security and the ability to make your own money and be financially secure

Being in sync with the rhythms of nature e.g. sleep wake cycles and circadian rhythms.

The ability to be fully focused and present in the now

The ability to be grounded

The ability to manifest all material needs.

Tribal relationships i.e. the family and everything affecting relationships within the family particularly the relationship with the parents

Sex at the most basic animal level e.g. lust, sex drive

Genetics, all of those traits we have inherited through the family gene pool which may also include personality traits or karmic issues within the family system

Nutrition

The need to exercise

Care of the environment/ Mother Earth.

Our connection to Nature

As you can see, a lot of things influence the health of this chakra! From my 20+ years working in the realms of exercise, energy healing, nutrition and lifestyle coaching, I would estimate that over 90% of the population have serious root chakra issues. The global crisis in the economy is like an outer reflection of the inner reality for the majority of individuals i.e., entrenched belief in lack, chronic fear around money and a complete lack of respect for the earth.

To find out how you fare with respect to root chakra health answer the following questionnaire with a true or false answer.

A. Physical Appearance

1. I am very overweight and or have a high level of body fat.

2. I am very underweight and would describe myself as skinny.

3. In proportion to the rest of my body my legs look very skinny.

4. I have a lot of fat on my legs.

5. I have no real muscle in my buttocks. In fact I could be described as a pancake butt.

6. I am not totally happy with how my body looks.

B. Health

1. I never seem to have enough energy to get through the day.

2. I am very reliant on coffee and stimulants to get going in the morning.

3. There is a history of heart disease in my family.

4. I seem to pick up every bug that's going.

5. Every year I take time off work due to illness.

6. I suffer from high or low blood pressure.

7. I do not train with weights.

8. I have been diagnosed with sarcopenia.

9. I have problems with my feet.

10. I have problems with my knees.

11. I have problems with my hips.

12. I have arthritis.

13. I have signs of high inflammation e.g. high cholesterol.

14. I have chronic muscle tension.

15. I suffer from constipation and /or diarrhoea.

16. I have been diagnosed with colitis or another colon disorder.

17. I suffer from frequent urination.

18. I suffer from stress urinary incontinence.

19. I have a very low libido or excessive libido.

20. I have erectile dysfunction.

21. I have osteoporosis or osteopenia.

C. Financial Security

1. I struggle to pay all of my bills every month.

2. I have a large overdraft or credit card debt.

3. I can't seem to control my spending and splurge on things I can't afford.

4. I have great difficulty turning my dreams into a reality.

5. I grew up in a household where there was a poverty consciousness.

6. I constantly worry about money.

7. I feel guilty if I buy something for myself.

D. Family

1. I have a very poor relationship with one of my parents.

2. I have a very poor relationship with both parents.

3. I never knew my parents.

4. I lost a parent at a young age.

5. I have a difficult relationship with one or more siblings.

6. I am estranged from my family.

7. I minimise contact with my family.

8. One or more family members no longer communicate with me.

E. Environmental Consciousness

1. I rarely spend time in nature.

2. I have no interest in gardening, plants or flowers.

3. I have no pets or I don't really care for animals.

4. I am not very environmentally aware. I rarely recycle and just use conventional cleaning products and personal care items.

5. The terms unprocessed food, locally sourced, seasonal and organic food do not have much meaning for me as I live off fast food and processed foods I get from a big supermarket or take away .

How did you Score?

If your total number of true statements were:

5 or less: you have low stress levels

10 or less you have medium stress levels

11 or more: you have high stress levels

So, now that you have an idea of how imbalanced your root chakra is, let's look at the ways in which we can support its healing.

Chapter 2

Nutritional Healing; The basics.

The foods that support your root chakra are also good for your body as a whole. Your body is a physical entity and the root chakra rules the physical plane. Your genetics and epigenetics (i.e., how the environment impacts the expression patterns of your genes) essentially dictate what foods are best for you.

What you have genetically speaking has been handed down to you from several generations. Since your genetic make-up doesn't alter much from one generation to the next, your ancestors diet is likely to be what's ideal for you. One of my mentors, Charles Poliquin, often states "We are cave men wearing business suits and carrying mobile phones". The world might look very different now to the cave man era but don't let all of that convenience food fool you. If your ancestors from thousands of years ago did not have access to that food, chances are it will do you more harm than good.

There are some principles that apply to everyone regardless of their genetic origins:

1. Eat a diet comprising of wholefoods that have not been tampered with in any way.

If in doubt ask yourself "Would a caveman have had access to this item?" E.g. Berries – Yes, Bagel – No . Steak – Yes, Chicken Mc Nuggets –No, Walnuts – Yes, M and M's –No, Water – Yes Red bull- No. Another of my favourite simplifications is "Don't eat anything that comes with an ingredients list" e.g., Chicken, Broccoli, almonds, Kale, Cherries, Flaxseed. None of the previous items comes with an ingredients list so you don't have to worry about additives and preservatives and extra sugar.

2. Eat Organic foods whenever possible.

There is a huge movement out there driven by commercial farming and other insidious interests that want to belittle the organic movement. If one considers the facts organic food is the way to go, from every conceivable angle. It's eco-logical. Logical in that it makes sense - sense for you and your family and sense for your environment. Caring for your environment does not constitute some new age hippie talk. We are the only animals that sully our nest so to speak. Trash and pollutants invariably end up in our bodies. The price you might pay could be liver disease, heart disease, cancer or many other potential disease outcomes. By eating organic food we reduce environmental pollution and thereby our own toxic load. One of the latest pieces of research shows much higher antioxidant level in organic food (up to 69% more) and less pesticide residues[1]. It has been estimated that your liver has to detoxify at least 800 chemicals per day. Do not add to this burden by buying non-organic foods. Non-organic foods are heavily sprayed with pesticides, fungicides and many other extremely toxic chemicals. Many people say they cannot afford organic food. In my estimation your food bill should be your most important health investment. It is funny how we find the money to buy wine, cigarettes, fashion and fancy cars, yet we baulk at the idea of investing in the nourishment of the vehicle of our entire life experience - our own bodies.

If you are genuinely strapped financially, you can minimise your exposure to pesticides in non-organic foods by employing some of the following tricks:

- Wash all fruits and vegetables in water and some apple cider vinegar. You can even buy solutions at the health food store to wash produce in.

- Foods that have to be peeled have less pesticide than thin skinned fruits.

- Limit your exposure to foods that have notoriously high levels of pesticide such as coffee, tea, apples, celery, strawberries, peaches, spinach, nectarine, grapes, sweet bell peppers, potatoes, blueberries, lettuce and kale.

Invest in organic meats whenever you can. Non-organic meats contain antibiotic residues. The animals are pumped with steroids to accelerate growth rate and in the USA it is legal to feed cattle cement dust. For more details on this read Jeremy Rifkin's 'Beyond Beef'.

For certain metabolic types (a system that classifies your body as one of 6 types depending on how it processes food) meat is essential to their wellbeing. The meat however, ideally, should be organic; even better if it's wild. Your minimum standard should be free range.

3. Increase the amount and variety of vegetables in your diet.

I have heard it said that if a nutritional convention were held, the only thing that the participants would agree on would be to eat more vegetables. The type of vegetables and the absolute amount will vary from one metabolic type to another, and from one individual to another. But as a basic principle "eat more vegetables" is sound. *Mark Houston*, MD, (Associate Clinical Professor of Medicine, Vanderbilt University), recommends at least 10 servings of vegetables and fruits a day (mostly vegetables) to reduce the risk of heart disease. Robert A. Rakowski, DC, CCN, states that it may take as much as 13 servings of vegetables and fruits a day to reduce cancer risk based on the latest research.

Why are vegetables so important?

They contain a range of vitamins, minerals, phytonutrients and fibre that are essential to health and wellbeing. Phytonutrients /Phytochemicals are a very broad class of chemical compounds coming exclusively from plants. They include:

- Phenolic compounds (i.e., carvacrol, which can be found in oregano and thyme) have strong antibacterial properties.

- Terpenes like lycopene which can be found in tomatoes. These have demonstrated strong anti-tumour and antioxidant properties.

- Betalains (i.e., betanin which gives beets their intense purple colour) have powerful antioxidant properties.

- Organosulphides (i.e., sulphorophane, which can be found in the brassica family of vegetables) have strong anti-tumour and anti-oestrogenic properties.

- Indoles (i.e., di-indoylmethane (DIM), which can be found in cabbage and kale) have powerful anti-aromatase capabilities.

There are literally thousands of phytochemicals. Only a small percentage of them have been studied in detail. These phytochemicals constitute very powerful medicine. In this modern era of disease, toxicity, obesity depression and despair we desperately need to harness the power of phytochemicals, vitamins and minerals. A nutrition protocol that only looks at weight loss via an equation to balance calories versus energy expenditure is a myopic one at best and a very dangerous unhealthy one at worst.

4. Fruit is Mother Nature's candy.

Fruits contain vitamins and minerals and those vital phytochemicals just discussed. It also contains high levels of sugar, hence its sweet taste and appeal. The sugar found in fruits is predominantly fructose. There is a dreadful misconception among certain groups, like the raw food movement and vegans, that the more fruit you eat the better. This however presents problems.

Fructose is a monosaccharide sugar which has an unusual property among sugars in that it has almost no impact upon insulin. For the most part, when you ingest a sugar (and there are several types of sugars) it stimulates a release of insulin from the pancreas. The insulin then ushers the sugar out of the bloodstream and into the body cells (muscle, liver or fat cells). Fructose however has almost no impact on insulin. Robert Crayon, Nutritionist, used to say that "Fructose is the guest who comes to dinner and never leaves". This is a big problem. If insulin is not secreted the fructose hangs around in your blood stream for a long time and causes a process known as glycation. In lay man's terms this is a type of caramelisation of your cells. It causes them to stick and clump together and is the very same process that causes diabetics to get gangrene. The average healthy person can cope with 30 grams of fructose a day (Source: Dr Georges Mouton, MD). A couch potato can handle 5 grams (this estimate comes from Olympic strength coach Charles Poliquin). Now if you eat one medium sized apple (3 inch diameter) you are ingesting 13.3 grams of fructose!

So everyone has to modify the amount of fruit they eat based on several factors:

    A. Your metabolic type (a system of eating for your genetics based on hundreds of questions screening how your body reacts to food, food preferences, physiological markers and psychological markers).

Sympathetics and Slow Oxidisers can handle more fruit than Parasympathetics and Fast Oxidisers.

You can find a Certified Metabolic Typing Advisor at: www.mt-advisors.info

B. Your innate insulin sensitivity.

Individuals are born with a genetic giftedness for insulin sensitivity or not. Persons with high insulin sensitivity have cells that respond optimally to insulin's signals, resulting in the distribution of carbs and sugars these individuals eat to their liver and muscle tissues. Those who lack insulin sensitivity have cells that don't respond optimally to insulin's signaling, which results in the distribution of carbs and sugars to the fat cells. These individuals get fat very quickly on a carb and sugar rich diet. Getting your biosignature tested is the quickest way to find out if you are insulin sensitive or not. You can find a certified Biosignature practioner in your area by looking here

http://www.poliquingroup.com/TrainerDirectory/FindaCoach.aspx

C. Your state of blood sugar regulation.

Individuals with really poor blood sugar regulation are described as diabetic. What must be understood is that diabetes is not an all or nothing phenomenon. Diabetes is simply the end zone of an ever escalating scale of poor blood sugar handling. Signs of poor blood sugar handling include sugar cravings, irritability if meals are missed, dizziness if a meal is late, extensive body fat around the waist and mood swings.

Poor blood sugar handling is known as dysglycemia. Your blood sugar could be too high (hyperglycaemia), too low (hypoglycaemia) or swing between the two (cortisol /Insulin see-saw).

If you have any of these problems and if you have anything less than a lean waistline you need to use fruit in small quantities if at all. Functional medical Doctor, Georges Mouton MD, recommends patients with diabetes and high uric acid levels to keep their daily fructose intake to around 15g per day. If you eat 6 dates you are already at 21.6 g of fructose!

D. Your current state of health.

Although the sugar found in fruit is presented in its natural state (i.e., combined with fibre and nutrients), this can still cause problems for some individuals. Cancer feeds on sugar, as does candida, and a variety of bacterial, fungal, yeast or mould infections. This is not something we would like to support in the body. Simply by cutting out all sources of sugar, many disease states and parasites can no longer thrive.

5. Protein; a must for all metabolic types.

The word protein comes from the Greek word *proteios* meaning "of first rank or first importance". In fact protein is considered essential to the human body. Not enough of it, or poor quality proteins lacking the essential amino acids (the building blocks of protein), lead to many health concerns that are very wide ranging. The most severe diseases of muscle wasting like Marasmus or Kwashiorkor are normally only observed in severely malnourished populations of the third world. In the western world, sarcopenia, or muscle wasting is very common among aging populations and can be mitigated to an extent with increased protein intake.

Protein is responsible for the growth and repair process of tissue which is happening on an ongoing basis. So individuals with compromised protein intake may have low muscle mass. Since muscle mass and its maintenance is the number 1 predictor of a person's lifespan (according to William Evans PhD and William Rosenberg, MD, professors of Nutrition and medicine at Tufts University), the importance of a diet rich in protein becomes apparent.

As well as promoting growth and repair, protein is very essential for detoxification. Most people associate detox with fruits and vegetables and vegan diets. While fruits and vegetables can provide valuable nutrients and fiber, they do not contain large amounts of protein. Amino acids like glutamine, lysine, taurine and carnitine bind onto toxins from phase I detoxification in the liver in a process known as amino acid conjugation to complete phase II. Funnily, the end products of phase I detox are often more toxic than the original toxins the body was trying to get rid of. It is imperative that the body has adequate access to a pool of amino acids to complete the phase II part of liver detox and enable the very toxic molecules to be released out of the body.

So, as an example, if you are on a vegetarian/vegan diet or juice fast, your levels of carnitine may be abysmal. If one consumes 100g of beef, they ingest 95mg of carnitine compared to a mere 0.195mg if they comsume 100g of asparagus (one of the highest plant sources of carnitine).

Taurine, another key player in amino acid conjugation, is virtually absent in vegetarian and vegan diets but is rich in meat and sea food diets.

6. Fats are essential for optimum health.

Like protein, fats are an essential component to every person's diet. Whether you are an Eskimo or a European, everyone would die on a diet of zero fats.

Some facts about fats in your body:

Your brain is about 66% Fat. Gives a whole new meaning to the term smart fats.

The myelin sheath covering your nerve cells is 70% fat.

Cell membranes are made up of about 50 % fats, a combination of phospholipids (lipids are a type of fat) and cholesterol which is another type of fat.

Cholesterol, which has been demonised by many, is essential to all human life. It is the raw material for the formation of hormones in the body and is a structural material constituting a high percentage of a cells membrane giving it appropriate sturdiness. Without cholesterol you would be completely infertile and have a non-existent libido. Fat of the land indeed.

One of the most visible signs of fatty acid deficiency is dry skin, brittle nails and hair.

The percentage of fat you need in the diet is dependent on your metabolic type. Low fat diets are not suitable for everyone.

Low fat diets can lead to depressed androgen levels and lead to muscle catabolism and difficulty in fat loss.

Low fat lies

"Most of us would have predicted that if we can get the population to change its fat intake... we would see a reduction in weight. Instead, we have seen the exact opposite."

Professor Harlan Onsrud, University of Maine

"We have found virtually no relationship between the percentage of calories from fat and any important health outcome. "

Professor Walter Willett of Harvard University, (arguably the most prestigious nutrition researcher of our time and lead author on both the Nurses' Health Study and the Health Professionals Follow-Up Study)

"Eat less fat and more carbohydrates may be the cause of the rampaging epidemic of obesity in America. "

Gary Taubes (science researcher and writer for the New York Times)

"For a large percentage of the population, perhaps 30 to 40 percent, low-fat diets are counterproductive," says Eleftheria Maratos-Flier, director of obesity research at Harvard's prestigious Joslin Diabetes Center. "They have the paradoxical effect of making people gain weight."

In a multi-year British study involving several thousand men, half were asked to reduce saturated fat and cholesterol in their diets, to stop smoking and to increase the amounts of unsaturated oils such as margarine and vegetable oils. After one year, those on the "good" diet had 100% more deaths than those on the "bad" diet[2].

Low fat diets are linked to depression. The father of the ultra-low fat diet Nathan Pritikin committed suicide.

What kind of fats do you need?

The body needs a broad fatty acid profile. Fatty acids are what fats are broken down into once digested (along with glycerol). Essential fats are ones the body can't make on its own. There are 2 of them; alpha-linolenic acid and linoleic acid. These are found from plant sources. The body then converts the plant form of the fatty acid into a form it can use. This creates EPA and DHA (eicosapentaenoic acid and docosahexaenoic acid) from ALA and Gamma linoleic acid from linoleic acid (LA).

The best source of essential fats.

Many people mistakenly believe that if they take flax or hempseed oil or some other commercially produced plant based oil that they have their essential fatty acid requirements covered. This could not be further from the truth. A diet high in LA can inhibit the conversion of ALA into EPA and DHA by as much as 40%. Many cofactors are required to make the conversion of ALA to EPA and DHA; these include vitamin C, B6, B3, zinc and magnesium. Practically everyone has low levels of at least one of these nutrients. Research also shows that less than 15% of ALA converts to EPA and less than 5% converts to DHA even when conditions are ideal.

In one study, supplementation with hemp seed oil for 12 weeks did not increase EPA and DHA at all and flaxseed supplementation only increased ALA[3].

High intakes of omega 6 fatty acids (largely from refined vegetable oils) can reduce the conversion of ALA to EPA and DHA by as much as 40-50%.

In people with diabetes and metabolic syndrome ,which is essentially a sliding scale of poor blood sugar handling, difficulties in converting ALA to EPA and DHA can arise as a result of dysfunction of enzymes needed in the conversion process [4].

In my practice, the vast majority of clients I see (over 90%) have some degree of blood sugar handling issues, at least until they get their nutrition and exercise programs sufficiently implemented. This is one of the many reasons why I never recommend plant based sources of essential fats.

One can get omega 3s by eating oily fish a few times a week but care is required not to heat to too high temperatures so as to minimise the damage to the sensitive EPA and DHA molecules that are rapidly oxidised (and thereby damaged).

The best option is to take an additional supplement of pure pharmaceutical grade fish oil at a dose of at least 1 teaspoon of fish oil per day as a base line. I use higher amounts of fish oils for limited periods of time with clients who have potentially been deficient in these fatty acids for years. Persons who have very high levels of body fat (over 20% for men and over 25% for women) can really benefit from such a tactic. It's not recommended for everyone however. Pregnant women need to seek individual guidance on any supplementation and, those who are scheduled for surgery are advised to stop taking fish oil supplements a few weeks before surgery to aid in blood clotting (fish oil reduces the stickiness/viscosity of the blood reducing its ability to clot as effectively). The 5ml baseline works well for most populations but if you are considering more then seek professional advice.

Fish oils can help mitigate most if not all disease conditions including, obesity, depression, Alzheimer's disease, multiple sclerosis, diabetes and heart disease.

"Almost everybody should be on omega 3 fatty acids for cardiovascular protection"

Dr Mark Huston MD

The Hypertension and Vascular Institute – Vanderbilt

Saturated fat- a health food?

For as long as almost anyone who has any interest in nutrition can remember, saturated fats have been demonised and vilified beyond redemption. The supposed bedrock of heart disease, it is usually preceded with the phrase "artery –clogging". According to the "experts" we have higher levels of heart disease and cancer because we are eating much more animal fats which are the principle source of saturated fats.

However for thousands of years food staples such as eggs, bacon fat, lard, suet, cream and the animal fats found in meats were consumed freely and heart disease was virtually unknown. In fact the first recorded heart attack was in 1921.

What we have seen from the early part of the 20th century onwards is a decrease in the consumption of butter and animal fats in general and an increase in the consumption of refined vegetable oils. Heart disease has continued to rise during this period. The notion that saturated fat is causative in high cholesterol levels and the formation of arterial plaque leading to heart disease has been disputed by many of the leading scientists in the world today:

"An almost endless number of observations and experiments have effectively falsified the hypothesis that dietary cholesterol and fats, and a high cholesterol level play a role in the causation of atherosclerosis and cardiovascular disease. The hypothesis is maintained

because allegedly supportive but insignificant findings, are inflated, and because most contradictory results are misinterpreted, misquoted or ignored. "[5]

Uffe Ravnskov PhD, MD

"How much total saturated fat do we need? During the 1970s, researchers from Canada found that animals fed rapeseed oil and canola oil developed heart lesions. This problem was corrected when they added saturated fat to the animals' diets. On the basis of this and other research, they ultimately determined that the diet should contain at least 25 percent of fat as saturated fat. Among the food fats that they tested, the one found to have the best proportion of saturated fat was lard, the very fat we are told to avoid under all circumstances!"

Mary G. Enig, PhD
(expert of international renown in the field of lipid biochemistry)

The research also shows that diets very low in fat and low in saturated fat can have a deleterious effect on testosterone levels. One study for example from "Journal of Steroid Biochemistry" in 1983 found that low-fat diets caused a large and significant drop in serum testosterone levels[6]. This makes sense on a biochemical level when we consider that testosterone is made out of a material called pregnenolone which in turn is produced from cholesterol. Many studies show increased saturated fat in the diet increases both LDL and HDL cholesterol. Very high fat diets give no additional benefit regarding optimising testosterone levels.

Monounsaturated fat

Another class of fats in nature are called monounsaturated. In chemistry terms the fatty acid chains have one double bond in practical terms these fatty acids come from sources such as nuts, olive oil, avocados and coconut oil. Diets rich in monounsaturates have been linked to a lower level of LDL cholesterol (although we now know that not all LDL cholesterol is bad just as not all HDL is good) Oleic acid, the principal monounsaturated fatty acid in olive oil has been linked to heart health by reducing hypertension.

Fats are a very concentrated source of calories so it's best to be mindful of portion control when having them. A small handful of nuts is a suitable portion for example. A quarter of an avocado will also be plenty. When it comes to oils think teaspoons at a time.

Gamma Linoleic Acid

Another fatty acid worth mentioning is the omega 6 fatty acid GLA. The best sources of this fatty acid include borage oil, blackcurrant seed oil and evening primrose oil. GLA has anti- inflammatory properties. Inflammation is the root cause of so many diseases like heart disease, diabetes, all types of arthritis, and Alzheimer's. It has been long used and recommended to women to enhance menstrual regularity and ease PMS symptoms. The GLA modulates key chemicals in the human body that regulate inflammation known as prostaglandins. GLA in conjunction with ALA has also been shown to reduce lower back pain and sciatica[7].

Many health food stores carry for example evening primrose oil in liquid form and it can be used to make salad dressings. Never cook with these delicate oils as they will be damaged by heat.

Conjugated Linoleic Acids

CLA has achieved some notoriety in the last decade or so with many studies touting it as an abdominal fat buster. CLA turns out to be not one molecule but a family of at least 28 different isomers of linoleic acid. The nature of the double bonds in CLA can be both cis and trans varieties. So here we have an example of a natural trans-fat that's actually healthy. Animals produce CLA with the trans conformations about the double bonds during the process of rumination. Wild meats have a higher concentration of CLA and therefore have greater health giving benefits. CLA has been shown in many studies to be anti-tumour and anti-cancer promoting. Some individuals get a reduction in belly fat when they supplement about 3.2 grams of this fatty acid daily[8]. The amount of fat lost is very modest but if you are looking to shave off 1 or 2 lbs from your midsection it may work for you.

Coconut Oil

There has been a lot of excitement over the last few years about the formerly maligned coconut oil. It was once feared due to its high saturated fat content. It's now known that the type of saturated fat in coconut oil is mostly Lauric acid, a medium chain triglyceride. MCTs are not handled the same way in the body as long chain triglycerides. They can be burned quickly for energy in the liver leading to more stable blood sugar and increased satiety. In fact they almost behave like a carbohydrate and are less likely to be stored as fat. Coconut oil has also been shown to be antiviral and antimicrobial. It boosts thyroid function and it is fantastic oil for cooking with due to a much higher smoke point. One word of caution! Make sure your coconut oil is not hydrogenated. You want the extra virgin kind. It's also very important that your oil is organic. Many of the tropical nations that produce the coconut oil use lots of pesticides so getting organic is a non-negotiable for this food.

Fats in Summary

The amount of fat that one needs in the diet as a percentage of overall calorie intake depends on the person's metabolic type which is in turn determined by the individuals' genetics and how those genetics express themselves in a given environment. What this means practically is that the amount of fat you need is dependent on genetics and how you are behaving on a day to day basis e.g. low activity level, high activity, aerobic exercise or anaerobic for example. Some people do better on a high fat diet e.g. fast oxidisers or protein types in the metabolic typing system. If this fast oxidiser gets really lean from an active lifestyle he or she will become more and more insulin sensitive and require more carbohydrate to stay in good energy production mode and ongoing fat loss mode. At this stage the amount of fat in the diet can be reduced to accommodate the increased energy supplied from the carbohydrate. The fatter you are the worse your insulin sensitivity and the better you do in general on a low carb diet at least till you get lean. Staying on a very low carb protocol long term can be deleterious to thyroid health.

The variety of fatty acids in the diet is key. Some saturated fats from meats, eggs and butter, some monounsaturated fats from nuts and olive oil, some medium chain fatty acids from coconut oil, the essential fats from EPA and DHA and some GLA. Getting a nice even spread of these for everyone is best. In an ideal world you would get a fatty acid profile tested from a blood test via a functional medical practitioner or nutritionist.

Going too low on the fats will eventually backfire on an individual. Your hormonal system will suffer and your appetite may be sky high (fats slow down the rate of digestion and increase satiety). Too much fat may tip you way over your caloric requirements for the day and will not give you any hormonal advantage.

Chapter 3

Specific foods to heal the foundation

The root chakra is represented by the colour red. The colour indicates the type of energy frequency we are dealing with. In nature, the colour of foods can steer us towards key nutrients that would benefit a given region of the body. The root chakra governs the muscles, bones and connective tissue so any nutrient that supports these structures supports the root chakra as a whole. This includes the heart which is also a muscle.

Red meat

Red meat has been demonised by vegan and vegetarian societies and some ill-informed nutritional advisors over the years. It has been blamed for cancer, obesity and heart disease. However, as is the case with many things in life, red meat has a lot to offer if approached with awareness.

Red meat is one of our key sources of saturated fat. Now that we know the many benefits of saturated fat, we need not fear it. Red meat gives a perfect amino acid profile making it a complete protein. In Chinese medicine it is considered a yang food or fire food, perfect for liberating energy. This makes red meat a great choice to start the day.

If your metabolism is functioning efficiently you should wake up hungry. Red meat is very satiating. The principle hormones associated with the root chakra (cortisol, adrenaline, pregnenalone, testosterone and DHEA) are all modified favourably with red meat. Many studies show that meat eaters have more favourable testosterone levels. Testosterone is made from DHEA.

Meat eating is strongly correlated with enhanced athletic performance, greater levels of strength and hypertrophy[1].

It is exceptionally rare to find someone with impressive muscular development who does not eat meat. Aside from the red meat testosterone connection , there are many reasons for this. Zinc, which is a very important mineral in muscle building and testosterone level maintenance, is found in high levels in meat and is also bioavailable(more readily absorbed into the bloodstream). Low zinc levels are correlated with low testosterone as well as impaired immune system and slow wound healing.

Red meat is an excellent source of iron and the form of iron it supplies is called heme iron. This form of iron is more easily absorbed than non- heme iron found in plants. Iron is necessary for the formation of red blood cells and lack of it leads to a form of anaemia. This will seriously impair energy production and hamper any athletic training.

Red meat reduces risk of depression in women. Researchers in Australia studied a group of 1000 women and they found that those who ate less than the recommended amount (3-4 palm sized servings per week) of lamb and beef were twice as likely to be diagnosed with the mental health disorders[2]. The lead author of this study, Professor Felice Jacka, specifically recommended grass fed beef due to its superior fatty acid profile (more omega 3 fatty acids present and less pro inflammatory omega 6).

Red meat is an excellent source of carnitine. Carnitine is a compound which helps shuttle fatty acids into the mitochondria(a sub unit of a cell involved in energy production) of the cells where they can be burned for energy. It is good for heart health, increased energy, reduction of fat mass and increase of lean body mass and treatment of peripheral vascular disease and diabetic neuropathy (university of Maryland medical centre). As I mentioned earlier red meat provides the best source of carnitine providing 95mg per 100g of beef steak. The highest plant source is avocado providing an abysmal 2mg per medium sized avocado.

Carnitine improves lean body mass (muscle) and heart function, one of our most important muscles. Thus, what is good for the muscular system is also good for the heart, and what supports the root chakra also supports the heart.

Grass fed red meat and wild red meats are rich in the fatty acid CLA. This has many health benefits, as stated earlier. In fact wild and grass fed meats are one of Natures' richest sources of CLA containing 3-5 times more CLA than their domestically grain fed counterparts.

Cherries

Cherries are another root chakra food. There has been an explosion of interest in this tasty red berry, particularly the tart cherries, as they have been shown to have a very powerful antioxidant capacity, reducing inflammation in the body. In one study of 20 women with osteoarthritis (an inflammatory condition), those who included tart cherry juice in their diets showed a significant reduction in symptoms in as little as 3 weeks[3].

Other studies show their application for reducing inflammation for athletes. Heavy training can increase inflammation in the muscles and joints. In many ways this is part of the natural training adaptation but if it is allowed to persist it can hamper recovery.

The anthocyanins (their red pigment) in cherries produce these anti-inflammatory effects.

They have also been shown to help reduce abdominal obesity. In the "Journal of Medicinal Food" October 26, 2009 rats that were fed tart cherry powder had significantly reduced levels of fat around the abdomen compared to rats who didn't, despite eating a similar diet with the same number of calories[4].

Research from the Centre for Biomarkers of Preventive Medicine, Doshisha University, Kyoto, Japan has shown that anthocyanins increase adiponectin (a cytokine) which has been shown to modulate diabetes and obesity in a positive way i.e. people lose fat easier[5]. Recent research has shown increased adiponectin levels in the body to be directly correlated in a causal way to increased insulin sensitivity[6,7].

With increased insulin sensitivity the body manages carbohydrate metabolism better.

Higher adiponectin levels facilitate the release of energy from fat cells more readily such that the body's metabolism is stimulated to increase fat burning. Higher adiponectin levels are also correlated with lower blood pressure and a reduction in atherosclerosis or hardening of the arteries.

Raspberries

Another amazing food for the root chakra is raspberries. They also stimulate increased adiponectin via the substance that gives them their distinctive smell – raspberry ketones. This could potentially stimulate a reduction of belly fat due to increased insulin sensitivity. Raspberries like cherries and all berries have powerful antioxidant capacity. An antioxidant quenches free radical reactions in the body. Free radicals are "rogue" molecules with an unpaired electron that can create havoc and destruction in the cells of the body.

Antioxidant levels in foods are measured according to a scale called the ORAC rating – Oxygen Radical Absorbance Capacity. 1 cup of raspberries has an ORAC rating of 6058, while sweet cherries come in at 4,873 (source Wikipedia). Raspberries are also high in fibre and low in sugar which makes them a dieters dream, with 100g yielding a whopping 8g of fibre and just over 5 grams of sugar. Raspberries are also a good source of vitamin C, a key nutrient for immune system health and adrenal gland health (the adrenals being the endocrine gland associated with the base /root chakra).

Raspberries also contain ellagic acid, a natural phenol antioxidant. It has been shown to protect the heart[8], kill cancer cells in a laboratory setting[9], and may assist in the detoxification of unfavourable compounds in the liver[10]. Ellagic acid has also been demonstrated to have potent anti-inflammatory effects[11]. In one study by Panchal et al from the European journal of Nutrition (April 2012) on ellagic acid the conclusion was very promising for the mitigation of the problems associated with a high fat and high carbohydrate diet[12]:

"Ellagic acid derived from nuts and fruits such as raspberries and pomegranates may provide a useful dietary supplement to decrease the characteristic changes in metabolism and in cardiac and hepatic structure and function induced by a high-carbohydrate, high-fat diet by suppressing oxidative stress and inflammation."

Rhubarb

Rhubarb is officially classified as a vegetable. . It has many health benefits including its laxative properties (attributable to its glycoside content), which can bring about natural relief for constipation.

Memorial Sloan- Kettering cancer centre lists Rhubarb as one of the foods that can help treat cancer and they site a number of research studies on their website to this effect.

Rhubarb has been shown to be good for the heart (again we see the heart root chakra connection) by lowering cholesterol and reducing blood pressure. It has been used successfully to treat pregnant women with hypertension.

Health care experts in Germany have been recommending an extract of rhubarb to treat hot flashes, a symptom of menopause, since the early 90s to very good effect.

A compound in Rhubarb, Piceatannol, has been shown by scientists to increase Nitrous Oxide (NO) in the body[13]. This is great for cardiovascular health and muscle building.

Rhubarb is also a very low calorie food with a low glycemic index. It's very low in sugar and has a decent serving of fibre. The downside is its very tart in taste and most people would like it sweetened. To keep it a low calorie healthy desert just stew it and sweeten with some stevia and add a little cinnamon. It's a guilt free treat that could work for you on so many levels.

Red Grapes and Red Wine

Most of us have heard of the "French Paradox" whereby the populous eats rich foods and drinks red wine daily and still has a lower risk of heart disease. Well one of the key reasons for this boils down to a compound called resveratrol. Study's on mice, which transfer well to humans, show that diets supplemented with resveratrol reduce fat gain during winter months where the animals normally gain fat.

Research on longevity continues to show that calorie reduced diets are the only known way of extending longevity. These low calorie semi starvation diets activate SIRT 1 genes which regulate cellular metabolism and longevity.

Resveratrol has been shown to mimic the effects of calorie restricted diets and has been shown to extend lifespan in insects, as well as vertebrates.

In many animal studies resveratrol has shown to be beneficial in treating cancers particularly skin and oesophageal tumors[14]. Research is ongoing in humans.

Drinking red wine has been demonstrated to have a cardio protective effect[15]. This is theorised to be a multiple pronged phenomenon of which resveratrol is part. According to the Mayo Clinic drinking red wine is correlated to lower LDL levels, reduced blood clotting, and protection against artery damage.

Resveratrol modulates oestrogen in the body. Resveratrol appears to work as an agonist or antagonist to oestrogen depending on the type of oestrogen in question. Some oestrogens provide protection and benefit to the body, others increase cancer risk.

Research from the University of Calabria in Italy has shown that resveratrol as an adjuvant therapy can help prevent the growth of malignant breast cancer tumours via blocking unfavourable oestrogens[16].

Life Extension magazine has reported that resveratrol can block prostate cancer at every stage of the disease and that it works by over a dozen anti-cancer mechanisms.

"One remarkable aspect of resveratrol is that it can be very toxic to cancer cells but does not harm healthy cells"

(LEF magazine April 2004).

Resveratrol inhibits the enzyme aromatase which converts testosterone into oestrogen. In order for men to remain healthy, virile, strong and confident the ratio of testosterone to oestrogen should be a minimum of 4:1 and better yet 8:1. These recommended ratios come from Dr Al Sears who uses resveratrol and other nutrients with his male clients to get the best hormonal profile for his patients.

Let it not be overlooked that females also have testosterone (one of our root chakra hormones) and if it drops very low or becomes aromatised they will also suffer the ill effects of this scenario; low sex drive, low motivation and confidence. Thus, females can also benefit from resveratrol's ratio boosting effects to favour a little more testosterone. Men who are aromatising(converting their testosterone to estrogen) strongly get man boobs (gynecomastia) and women get "side boobs" or that annoying fat at the point where the upper chest meets the arm pit. Even women as slim as Victoria Beckam have allegedly reported complaining of this. No amount of dieting will get rid of this but hormone optimisation via nutrition can!

Cranberries

Cranberries are another nutrient of the root chakra. One of the signs that the root chakra is out of whack is that there is systemic inflammation in the body. Inflammation is like the body is "on fire". The Latin origin means to set alight. Diseases linked to inflammation include arthritis, obesity, heart disease, brain disorders like Alzheimer's and digestive disorders like ulcerative colitis. Red, the colour of the root chakra, is also the colour associated with inflammation.

The compounds in cranberries that give them the red colour are called anthocyanins. These act as antioxidants to counteract inflammation:

"It seems small amounts of these phytochemicals find their way from plant foods, like cranberries, into our cells, and then direct cells to reduce our inflammatory reactions."

Jeffrey Blumberg Tufts University

Cranberries have also been shown to combat bacterial infections like urinary tract infection[17] and gum disease[18]. It would appear that something in the cranberries causes an anti-adhesion affect that stops bacteria sticking to cells.

Researchers at Cornell University have shown that cranberries help prevent the oxidation of LDL cholesterol and so help reduce heart disease[19]. They also help the liver absorb LDL more effectively which is then converted into bile which assists in the digestion of fats among other roles.

Goji Berries

Certain types of sugar molecules found in Goji berries have been shown to inhibit prostate cancer in animal studies[20] (university of Hong Kong)

In Chinese medicine the plant is revered as a longevity enhancer.

Research from Zhejiang University of Technology, China has shown that goji berries can increase muscular endurance by up to 50% [21].

Goji Berries contain betaine which lowers homocysteine (a marker of inflammation). They also contain beta-sitosterol, a plant sterol, which is believed to be the compound responsible for many of gojis health benefits including the lowering of LDL cholesterol.

Plant sterols have also been shown to mitigate the stress response by lowering cortisol and stimulating an increase in DHEA. DHEA is one of the sex hormones that can go on to produce testosterone. In one study on marathon runners those who received plant sterols as a supplement had better immune function, lower cortisol output, less markers of inflammation and an increase in DHEA[22].

Tomatoes

Tomatoes are botanically classed as fruits and belong to the nightshade family. Tomato based products may have a role in the prevention of prostate cancer[23]. In another study it was found that the more carotenoids the individual consumed, lycopene being one of them, the lesser the risk of prostate cancer[24]. In the Journal of the national cancer institute a study titled: "A Prospective Study of Tomato Products, Lycopene, and Prostate Cancer Risk" took a look at several other studies on the lycopene prostate cancer link and concluded that the consumption of tomato based products did have a significant impact on reduction of prostate cancer risk[25].

It should also be noted that cooking tomatoes increases the bioavailability of the lycopene significantly[26].

As well as containing lycopene tomatoes have a vast array of other nutrients to influence the base chakra in a favourable way. They contain vitamin C, which is very important for adrenal health, a key gland associated with the root chakra. Other nutrients that support the adrenals that are found in tomatoes include Vitamin B6, thiamine, niacin and a substantial source of potassium (with 1 cup of cherry tomatoes providing 353mg of Potassium) – (nutritiondata.self.com)

Tomatoes support bone health due to their vitamin K and calcium content. The root chakra is the prime driver of muscle, bone and connective tissue health. The root chakra supports you from below as we pull energy and chi from Mother Earth. In practical terms, the "fruits of the earth" allow us to replenish our chi daily. The musculoskeletal system supports our entire physical structure.

Exercising generates free radicals (rogue molecules with unpaired electrons that are highly unstable and reactive), which can damage your cells. To a certain extent, this is necessary to break the muscle down (in bodybuilding for example). What's important is that the tissues can recover from such free radical damage and get stronger and fitter in the process.

This recovery process is facilitated in part by the foods you eat. Scientists at Stockholm University showed a remarkable capacity of tomato juice at a dose of 150ml daily(yielding 15mg of lycopene in addition to other phytonutrients) to effectively reduce significantly one of the markers of DNA damage[27].

Tomatoes have been somewhat maligned as being part of the nightshade family of plants. These plants have been blamed for arthritis, migraine and osteoporosis but all of these concerns would appear to be anecdotal. In Best

Health Magazine (Canada) Sep 2009 a number of experts were interviewed about the potential hazards of nightshades. In every case no scientific evidence was found to support the theory that nightshades are actually responsible for the conditions mentioned.

"I'm not aware of any studies in peer-reviewed journals that prove or disprove that they (nightshade vegetables) affect arthritis. There are a lot of references to it, but the evidence is mostly anecdotal."

Mark Erwin, an assistant professor of orthopaedic surgery at the University of Toronto.

It should also be noted that cooking the tomatoes reduces the alkaloid levels (the chemicals suspected to potentially cause a problem) by half.

Each individual is so unique. If you suspect the nightshades are causing your problems, then get some food intolerance testing done. Sometimes the power of suggestion can create a placebo effect whereby a person has a problem with a food because they believe it is a problem. The easiest way to tackle the issue is to eliminate all nightshades for a period of 2-3 weeks and then reintroduce one at a time leaving 3 days between each new introduction. If the symptoms return then that food might not be for you.

Choosing the right foods for you

As you can see there are many foods that will support the root chakra. The trick is to get a combination that works for you. Working with a metabolic typing assessment is a great start. You can find an advisor to work with here: www.mt-advisors.info . Many advisors will work over the phone or internet. Some people work well eating red meat once a week or once every two weeks. Some people (like fast oxidisers) eat red meat several times a week. Those metabolic types that do really well on red meat are also usually engaged in heavy weight training. The take home message is that what work's for you may not work for someone else. It's very individualistic, and should be tailored according to your body and how it responds.

Chapter 4

Supplements to support the foundation

The root chakra governs the musculoskeletal structure: muscle, bone and connective tissue. The endocrine glands associated with this chakra are the testes and the adrenals. In this section I will look at supplements in addition to your baseline nutritional plan that you may like to consider to give yourself extra support. As with all other aspects pertaining to health, like exercise and nutrition, each individual's requirements are unique to them. The guide here is not intended as a definitive individual prescription. Ideally you would work with a nutritional advisor, functional medical doctor, naturopath or applied kineseologist to customise your plan.

Whey protein

Post work out recovery

For those who are lifting weights regularly, something which I would highly recommend, whey protein makes a great addition to your recovery plan. In the post workout window your cortisol levels (a stress hormone) are elevated. Your muscles are screaming for nutrients. This is one of the only times that I recommend a liquid meal. After the workout we want to get nutrients into the muscle cells as quickly as possible. A liquid meal is digested way faster than a solid one and in the post workout window this is highly desirable.

Whey contains the full complement of essential amino acids. *Whey protein* is a rich natural *source of BCAAs* (Isoleucine, Leucine and Valine); in fact it's one of the richest sources of BCAAs. These amino acids facilitate recovery, support strength development, increase endurance and facilitate a better testosterone/cortisol ratio.

Detoxification and immune system support

Whey not only helps one recover from exercise, it is also a potent facilitator of detoxification and a booster of the immune system.

Whey protein is rich in cysteine, glutamic acid and glycine which are all precursors to glutathione, one of the body's most potent antioxidants and detoxifiers. People who are chronically stressed have typically low glutathione levels. This sets them up for poor immune function and vulnerability to bacterial and viral infections. Anybody who is immune compromised (like cancer and AIDS patients) can really benefit from whey.

Weight loss

Whey has also been shown to be a friend of those trying to lose weight. In one study participants who took a whey drink before breakfast and dinner ended up losing more body fat and preserving more lean body mass[1]. Whey supports weight loss by satisfying appetite, supporting serotonin production and modulating the stress response.

Quality of whey

The quality of the whey is very important. The best sources come from New Zealand and are uncontaminated with antibiotics. The whey also comes from cows that are grass fed, which makes their milk even healthier, and contain higher levels of immunoglobulins (these are a range of special proteins which include beta-lactoglobulin, glycomacropeptide, bovine serum albumin, IgG and lactoferrin).

Some types of whey do not contain these immunoglobulins because they have been processed at an unsuitable temperature and the proteins have become denatured.

Which whey is best for me?

Whey isolate is most suitable for those with dairy allergies. Whey concentrate is fine for those who do not react badly to dairy. Whey hydrosylate is a hydrolysed form of whey isolate and requires minimal digestion but the taste leaves a lot to be desired. Make sure your whey is un-denatured and does not contain any additional sugars.

Vitamin C

Many animals can synthesise vitamin c on their own. Human beings are one of the few species that cannot synthesise it and hence it is an essential nutrient that must be ingested regularly from food or supplemental form.

At the most basic level, vitamin C deficiency leads to a disease called scurvy. This is extremely rare in developed countries. Vitamin C functions as an electron donor for many reactions in the human body and hence is an important antioxidant. Vitamin C facilitates the absorption of iron.

Vitamin C is critically important to mitigate the stress response. The adrenal glands, which are two small endocrine glands sitting on top of the kidneys, contain the bodies highest concentration of vitamin C in the body, roughly 100 times blood plasma levels. The adrenals secrete vitamin C as part of the stress response[2].

One study from the University of Wisconsin showed that a 500 mg dose of vitamin C improved endurance in obese subjects[3]. Anywhere between 1 and 3 grams a day can be used or to bowel tolerance (if you get loose stools you are taking too much!) You may need the higher end of the scale if you have high stress levels or a high training volume or you are a smoker.

B vitamins

The B vitamins are required for the production of adrenal hormones in conjunction with vitamin C. So the more stressed we are, the more we burn up B vitamins. One of the many forms of stress the body is exposed to is toxicity. The body requires many B vitamins, particularly B6, B9 and B12 to detoxify poisonous compounds from our bodies.

Vitamin B5 is known as the "anti-stress" vitamin. It is also critical to adrenal health. A derivative of vitamin B5 is called Panthethine. Vitamin B5 goes through 5 steps to become Co enzyme A, a key energy broker molecule in the body. Panthethine just goes through one step. This is very useful for those who are already stressed, compromised and fatigued, as metabolic processes become more inefficient with stress.

Panthethine specifically has been shown to support the formation of a compound called brain-derived neurotrophic factor which can regenerate the brain and support overall nervous system health. When we are being stressed by another person we have the expression "he/she is getting on my nerves" So if we can calm the nervous system, our overall system will be less stressed.

Branched chain amino acids

The root chakra governs muscle, bone and connective tissue so any nutrient, herb or food that supports these elements will also support the root chakra and by

When potassium levels are decreased and sodium levels are increased (in conjunction with chloride values) it's a marker for hyper-adrenal function. When the potassium levels are increased and the sodium levels are decreased this is a marker (in conjunction with chloride values) of hypo-adrenal function.

Electrolyte balance is critical for many reasons, most notably cellular hydration. Many people are under the illusion that just drinking enough water is enough. In many cases it is not. If the person's adrenal health is compromised, their electrolyte balance can be so skewed that the body cannot hydrate its cells correctly.

A charge is required to get fluids into and out of the cells. This charge is provided by the electrolyte minerals. Poor electrolyte balance can lead to either high or low blood pressure as the fluid and hydration levels of the body have a massive influence on blood pressure.

So if you are not eating a diet rich in large quantities of vegetables with a modest amount of fruit (compatible with your metabolic type and hormonal health) it's likely you are not getting enough of these key minerals. Even if you are eating the appropriate amount of fruits and vegetables, you may still be deficient due to the poor mineralisation of our modern soils.

The more stressed you are the more you deplete your minerals. If you wish to supplement with electrolytes then get a formula that does not come in the form of a sports drink with sugars. Get the pure minerals with nothing else added.

Chapter 5

Stretches for the foundation

The muscle groups that I have designated to the root chakra were selected based on their location, function and properties. For the purpose of this section I will first identify the key muscle groups that assist base chakra function.

Muscle Groups

Feet/ankles

Shins

Calves

Hamstrings

Buttocks

Groin

I have designated the quadriceps as a second chakra muscle group for a variety of reasons.

Feet, Ankles, Shins and Calves.

Foot mobiliser

Point the toe like a gymnast, inhale, and then exhale to pull toes back towards the shin 8-10 times. You can also reverse the breathing pattern. Inhalation supports the lengthening of the muscle. Follow this with circles of the foot clockwise and anti-clockwise about 6 each way.

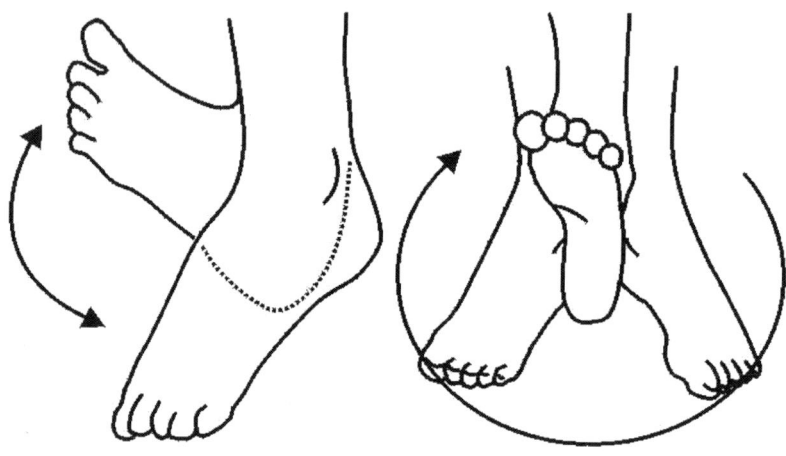

Shin and front of foot stretch

Sit back on your heels with front of foot flat on the floor. You can make the exercise more challenging by walking the hands back behind the feet and supporting some weight in the hands so as to protect the low back. You can stay in the position for 15 seconds then rock out of the deep stretch for a bit before going back into it again. Repeat at least 4 times.

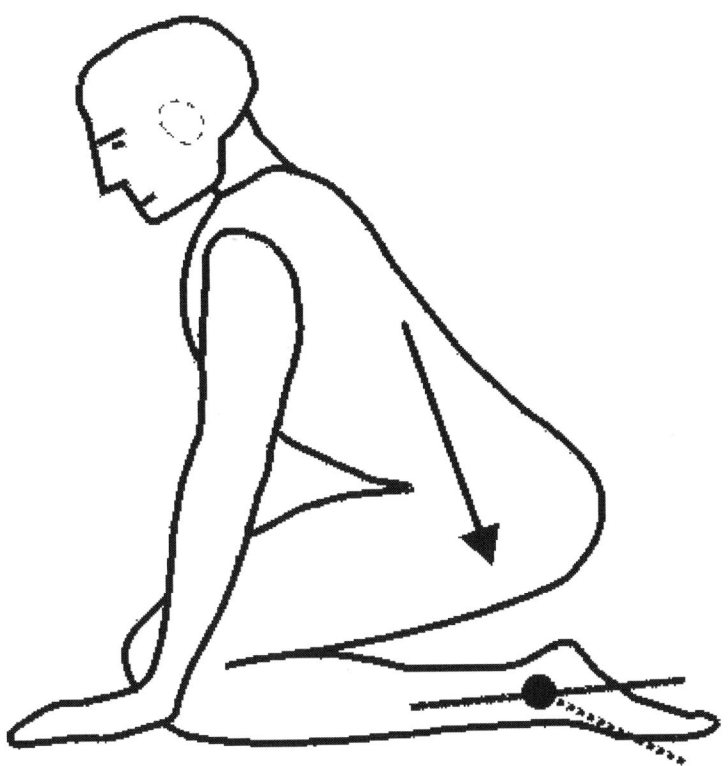

Plantar fascia stretch

Get into position like the last exercise sitting on heels only this time instead of the front of the foot flat bend the toes and put the weight on the balls of the feet. Lean back supporting with the hands to the degree required to feel the stretch. Some people will feel a stretch immediately as they are so tight. Stay in the deep stretch for 15 seconds, adjust body weight forward to reduce the stretch for a break and then lean back into the stretched position again. Repeat 4 times in total.

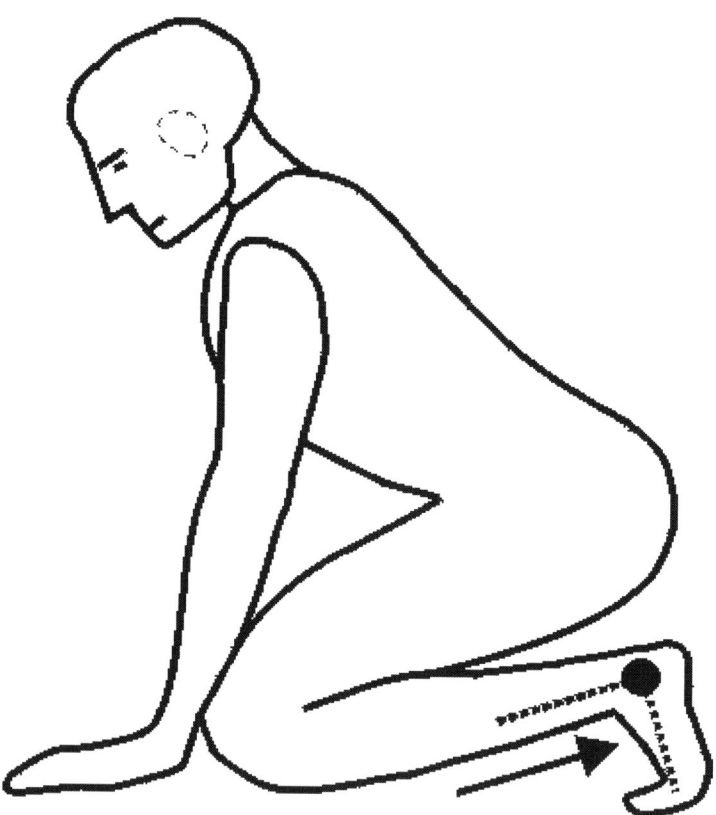

Ankle and Calf mobilisation and stretch

Stand on the last step of a stairwell or on a low step in a squat rack holding on securely. Start with balls of foot on edge of the step with heels over the edge. Start treading the heels over the edge deeply in an alternating fashion bending the knees appropriately to achieve the range of motion. Do this for 30-60 seconds. Then stop, drop down both heels and hold the stretch for 15 seconds. Then switch to one side at a time. Alternate between sides till you do 4 reps each side. Now repeat the last exercise with a 15-20 degree bend in the knee which will shift the stretch further up the calf. This series mobilises all of the calf musculature and the ankles.

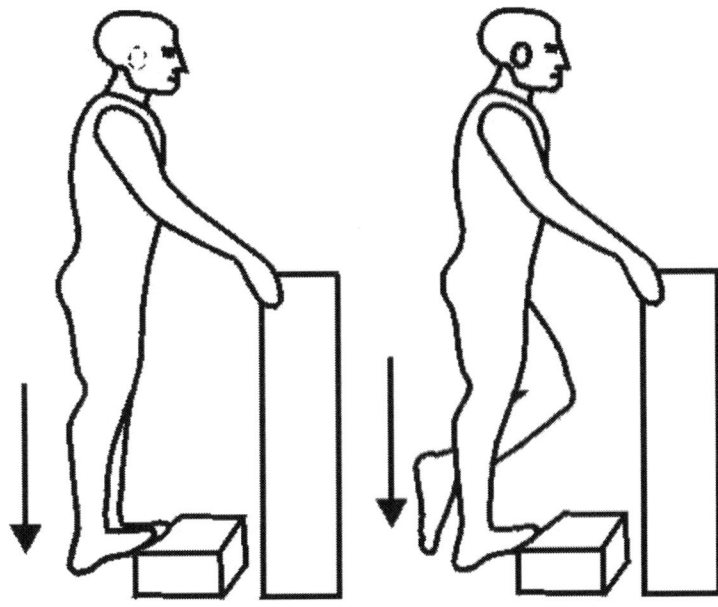

Calf and ankle wall stretch

Stand on one foot and place other foot against a wall. The ball of the foot is on the wall and the heel of the foot is on the ground. Lean into the wall while at the same time getting the hips to move towards the wall in unison. You can dynamically move in and out a few times then stay 15 seconds. Move dynamically again and stay another 15 seconds. Repeat this up to 4 times.

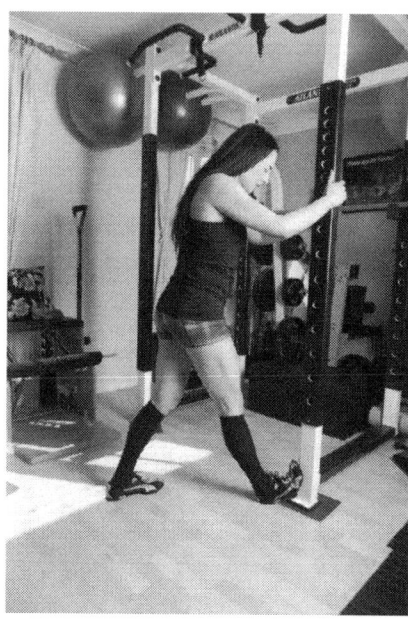 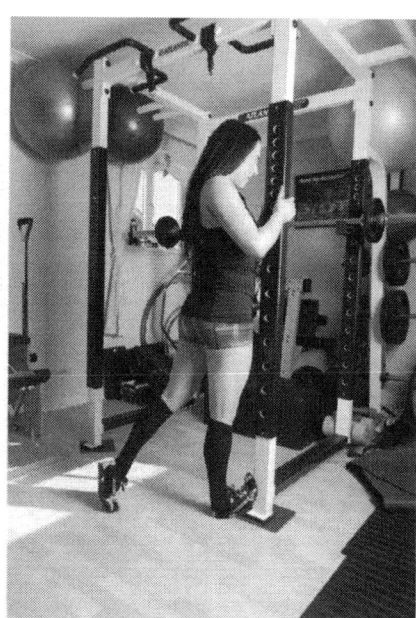

Plantar fascia stretch

Sit tall on a cushion if required to optimise a neutral pelvic position right up on the sits/sitz bones (these are the bony parts at the base of your pelvis technically called ischial tuberosities). Hook a towel around ball of the foot. Press ball of foot into towel at 10% effort for 8 seconds. Release and pull toes back towards shins with towel. Press again for 8 seconds and release. Repeat this 1-2 more times and stay for 15 seconds in the end range breathing smoothly throughout.

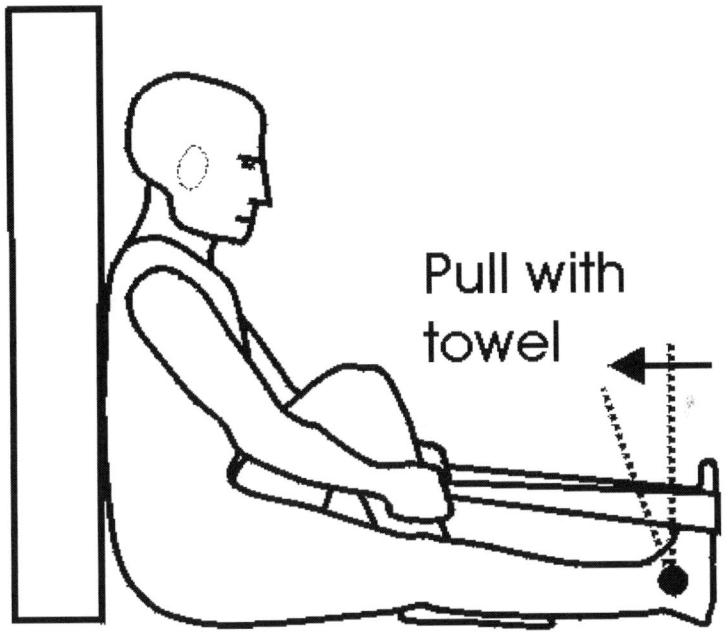

Hamstrings

Waiters Bow stretch

Stand with the legs hip distance apart. Slide the hands down the thighs initiating the move with a backward displacement of the hips. Tip the pelvis forward as if it were a bucket of water that you are emptying by tipping it forward. Keep the tailbone lifting and keep a neutral lumbar curve (a little dip in the lower back). Ideally you should be able to get down to a point where the finger tips touch the knees. Don't force this at the expense of losing the lumbar curve. Keep knees locked for the stretch. Stay in position for 15 seconds, bend knees and press up out of stretch. Slide down again and repeat process 3-4 more times.

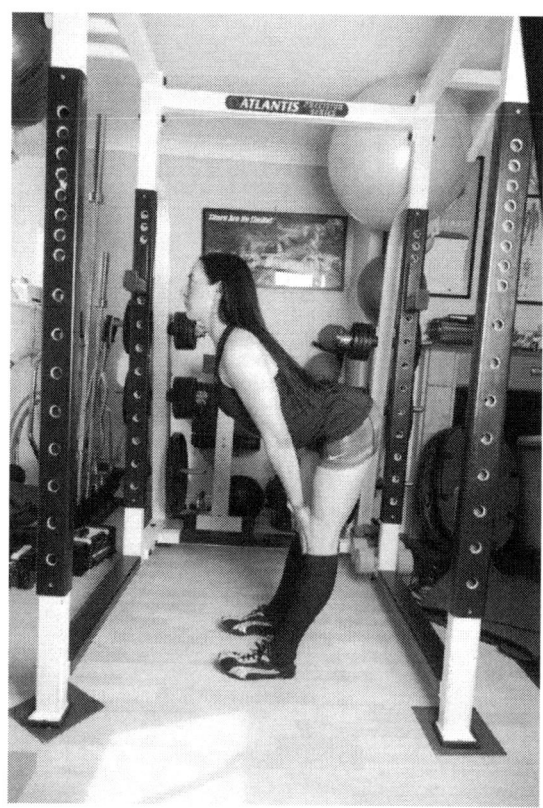

Supine band assisted stretch.

I learned this multi planar hamstring stretch from one of my many internships with Charles Poliquin. You can use a yoga strap for this or the belt on a bath robe, even a towel if you are stuck. Lay on your back with a small towel under it rolled up to support your lumbar curve. Wrap the band around your lower calf. The other leg is bent, foot on the floor for support. Press the leg into the band until you feel the hamstring contract. Hold the contraction for 8 seconds. Release the tension and immediately move into a deeper stretch by pulling the band closer to your body. Repeat the contract /relax move leg closer to your body 3-4 more times. Then stay in the peak stretch for 15 seconds breathing deeply and relaxing into the stretch. The effects of the stretch can be spread to all aspects of the hamstrings by repeating the sequence with the leg out to the side of the body at right angles and a final time by crossing the leg over the midline of the body. This way all regions of the hamstrings are hit effectively.

Supine Band Assisted Stretch in 3 Planes

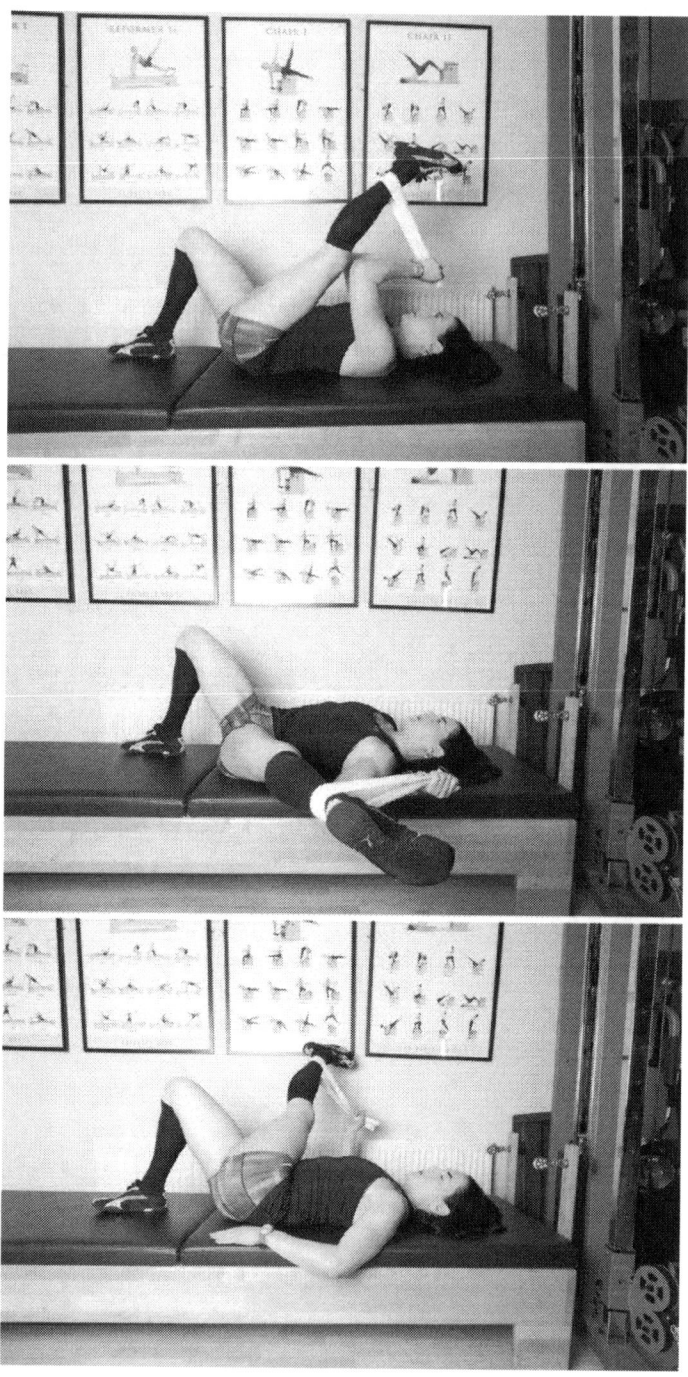

Seated hamstring stretch unilateral

You can prop yourself up on a towel for this one to try and get your pelvis nice and upright sitting up on the sits bones. Straighten one leg and place other foot tucked in beside the knee of the straight leg, knee out to side. Stay tall on the sits bones and hinge at the hips as opposed to folding at the waist. Slide hands down the straight leg as far as you can without rounding the lower back. Hold position for 15 seconds, slide up and repeat after a few seconds. Do it at least 4 times then do the other side. If one side is tighter than the other do the tight side first, then the other side, then the tighter side again.

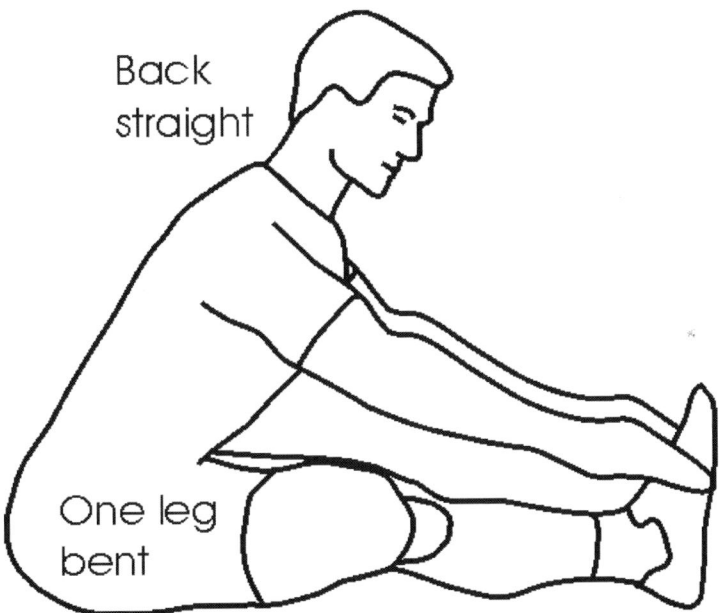

Bilateral seated hamstring stretch.

This stretch begins in the same position as the last sitting on the floor with a little folded towel under the buttocks to optimise pelvic position where necessary. Both legs are outstretched in a wide "V". Tip the pelvis forward as if you were emptying a bucket of water. Support the upper body with your hands. Walk them forward in front of you on the floor while simultaneously tipping the pelvis forward as if you are emptying a bucket of water. Keep the tail bone lifting. You are looking to feel the stretch at the point where the hamstrings meet the buttocks. Stay in the position head on for 15 seconds. Walk hands over to one side. Stay there 15 seconds. Walk hands to the other leg and hold 15 seconds. Go through this centre, side sequence a few times and at the end slide legs together, hinge forward and hold for 15 seconds.

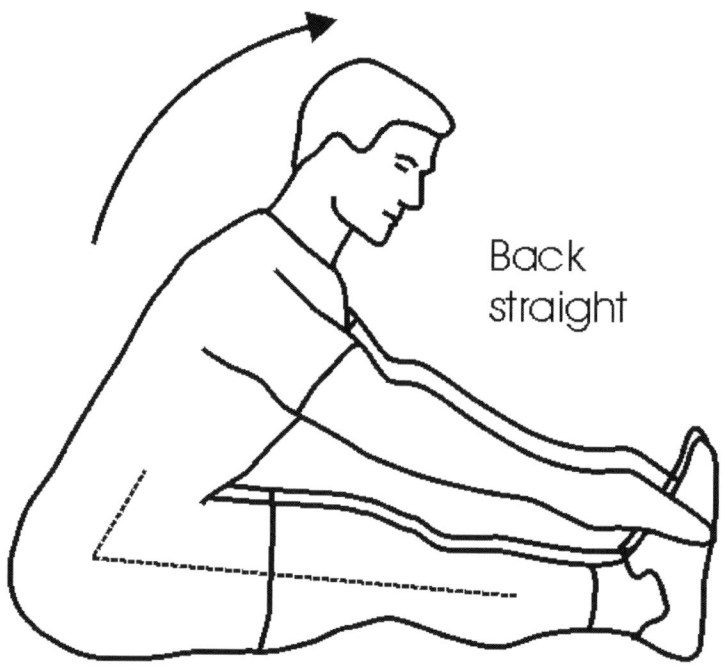

Bilateral Hamstring Stretch

Buttocks

Supine stretch

Lay on the back and cross one leg over the other. The shin of one leg is resting on the thigh of the other. Clasp behind the thigh that is perpendicular to the floor. Now hug that clasped thigh into the chest for 15 seconds. Now circle it clockwise 6-8 times and anti-clockwise 6-8 times. Repeat on the other side.

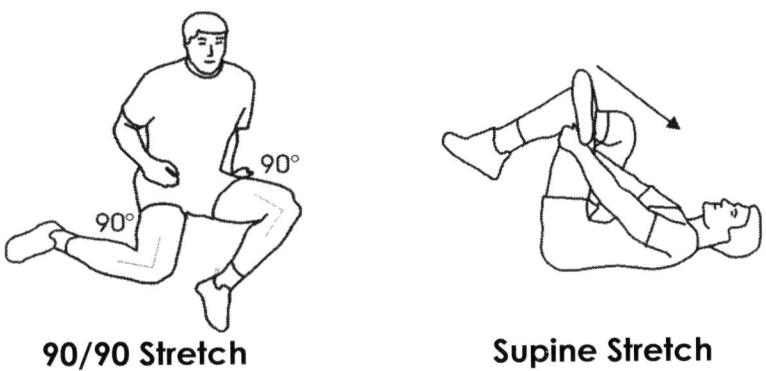

90/90 Stretch   **Supine Stretch**

90/90 buttock stretch and mobilisation

This exercise is a combination of two exercises. I learned the mobilisation part from Ann and Chris Frederick and the second part from Paul Chek.

Get into the 90/90 position as shown in the diagram. Start the mobilising portion of the exercise by diving your head and upper body down and over the front thigh. Lift the chin and come back up to the starting position. Repeat this dive and return to start position in a wave like motion 6-10 times, hands supporting on the floor on each side. Now go back to start position with the spine upright. Press the front shin into the floor at 10% effort for 8 seconds. Release the pressure and hinge at the hip as you lower the chest down a bit, keeping neutral spine. Repeat this contract/relax and move process till you go as deep as you can. Stay in the final position for 15 seconds and breath. Place hands on ground on either side of the body to support both mobilisation phase and contract relax sequence.

The lizard stretch

The introductory level of this stretch is fairly doable by everyone. The advanced version is a big progression. Take a large step forward and place hands on floor straddling the front knee or (my preference) two hands on same side. Sink the butt cheek of the front leg as deep as possible with most of weight on front heel. Stay 15 seconds then mobilise the leg forward and back for 15 seconds before dropping to deepest position again. Repeat this process over and back, deep drop down to dynamic movement about 4 times. Do the other side. Always do a tighter side first and repeat it again after stretching the not so tight side if you have an imbalance. The advance version of this exercise places the forearms on the floor on the inside of the forward leg. That's a much deeper stretch and one has to build up to it but it is an amazing glute/buttock stretch!

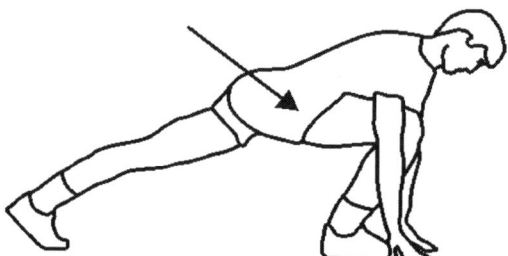

The lizard stretch

Bilateral seated buttock stretch

In this exercise you get to hit the buttocks in a different region again. This is the secret of good and effective stretching. We target the muscle group at multiple angles. Start by sitting on the floor cross legged. Hinge at hips while reaching arms up to lift up out of your sits bones. Now reach hands to floor (or elbows as in the picture, I prefer the hands to floor). Walk the finger tips out till you feel a nice stretch in the sides of the buttocks. Stay for 15 seconds and see can you walk the hands out a little more. In between each "walk out" with the hands we can create a contract relax effect by bilaterally pressing the knees laterally toward the floor before releasing them and moving forward again. At no stage should one feel any discomfort in the knee ligaments. Some individuals will also feel a subtle stretch in the lower back. This is fine as long as you maintain support of the lower back with hand contact on the floor in front.

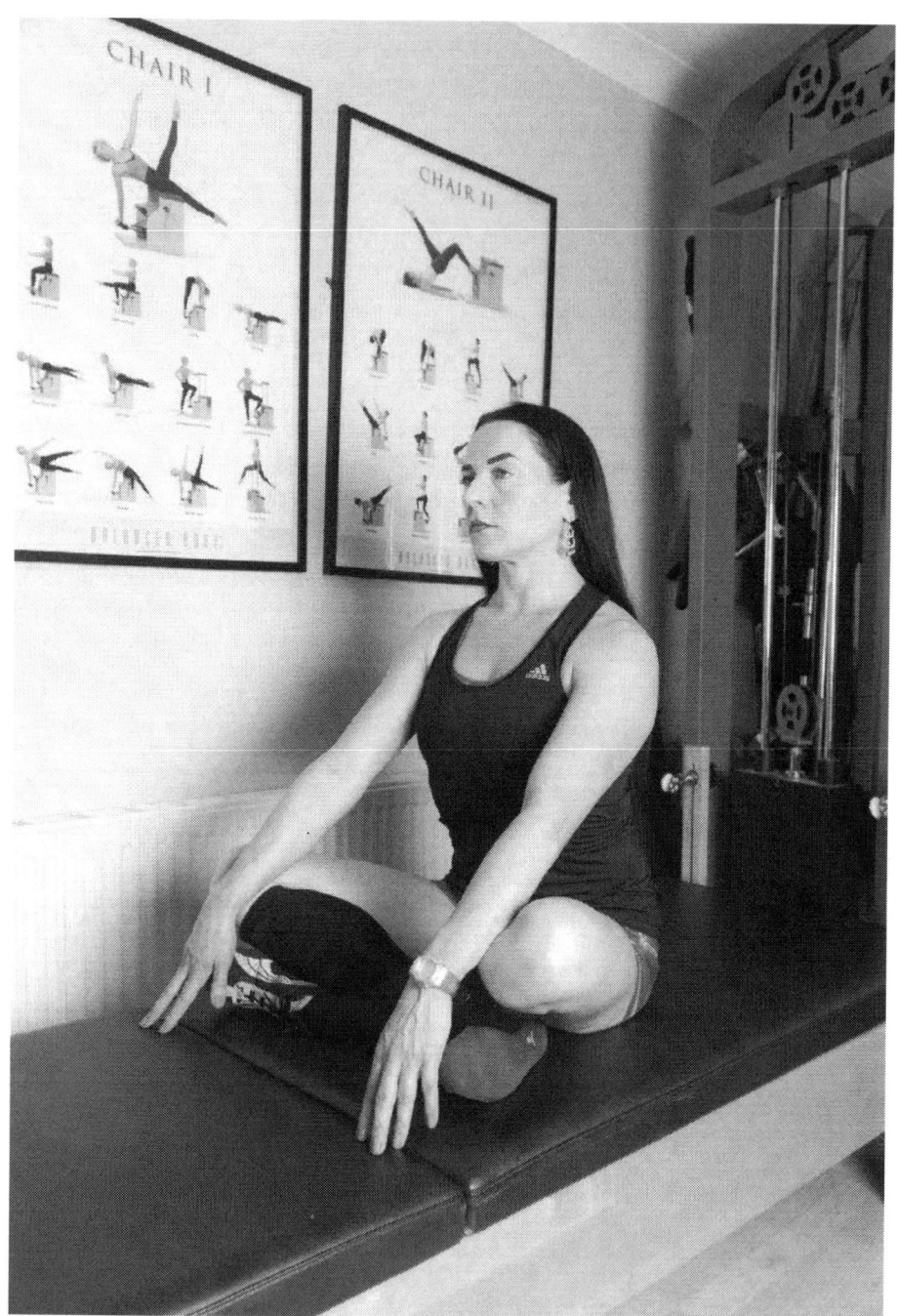

Starting position bilateral buttock stretch

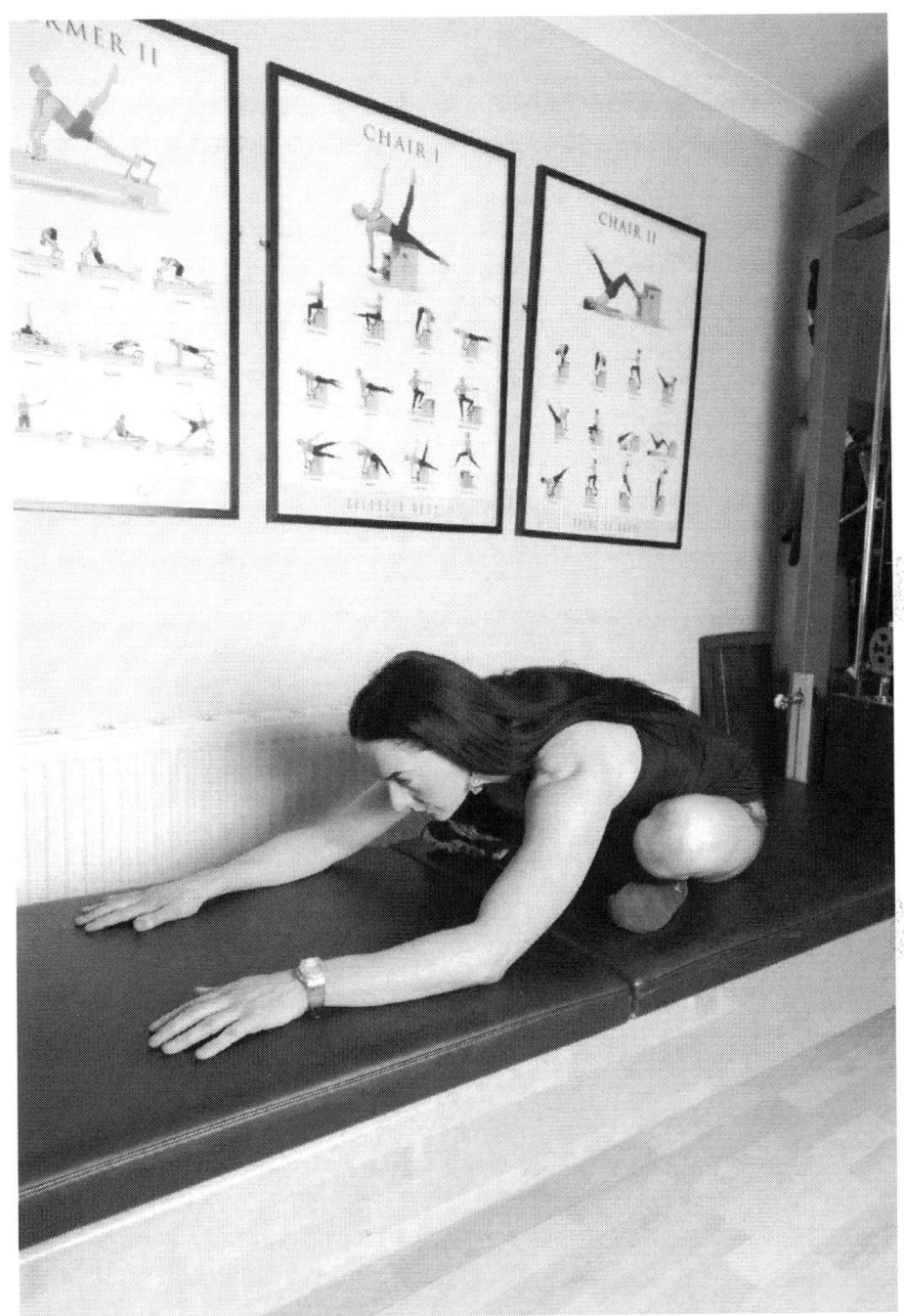

Finishing Position Bilateral Buttock Stretch

Groin

Seated Groin Stretch

Sit nice and tall on the sits bones. Inhale and press on inner thighs close to knees at 10% for 8 seconds. Release and immediately press thighs further apart. Repeat the contract/relax cycle 3-4 more times and stay in the maximally stretched position for 15 seconds. Keep a conscious engagement of your pelvic floor by squeezing the muscles that control bladder and bowel. This will make it easier to release the groin musculature.

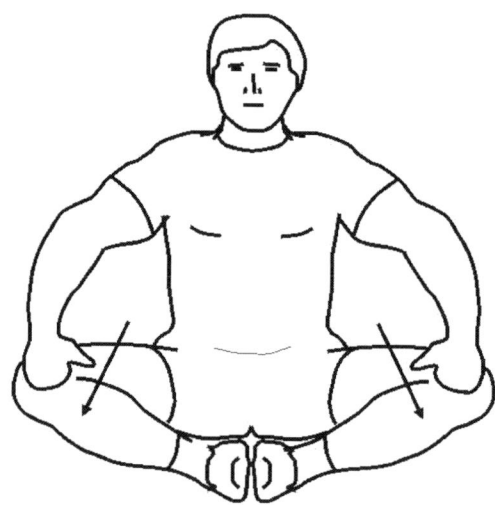

Prone groin stretch

This is another exercise I learned from Paul Chek during one of my many internships with his institute. This time get on to your mat, stomach downward, knees spread wide and bent. Support upper body with hands. Now gently press knees into floor (make sure you are on a soft mat) at about 5-10% effort. Hold this for about 8 seconds, relax and slide the knees slightly wider. Now walk hands forward a few inches and repeat this. Walk the hands a little forward again and repeat. Finally lower your body down to the forearms and hold the position for about 15 seconds.

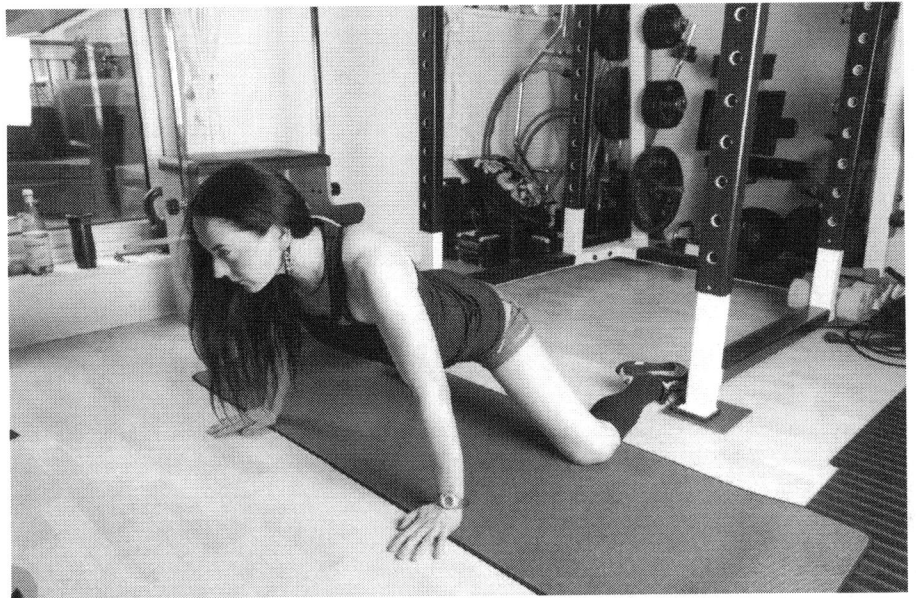
Position 1 Prone Groin Stretch

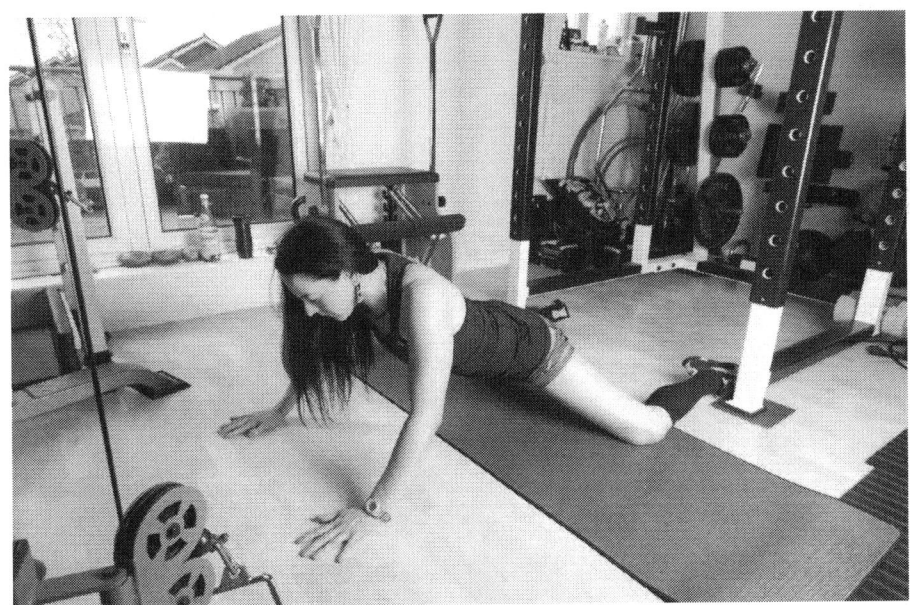
Position 2 Prone Groin stretch

Chapter 6

Corrective Exercises

In this section I will deal with some basic corrective exercises that will work the muscles of the root chakra. Most of them will focus on isolation exercises to really target inhibited or weak areas. There will also be some compound exercises that work multiple muscle groups and joints. Before one can perform a compound movement well all the muscles required should be able to fire well. If you have strength or stability deficits, due to weak muscle groups, performing a good squat through appropriate range with good form becomes almost impossible. Getting assessed with a trainer, qualified and experienced in this area, will allow you to identify your weak muscle groups and target them. This process will save you years of wasted time in the gym and substantially reduce your risk of injury and back problems.

The exercises I will cover will include exercises for:

1. **The feet**
2. **Calves and Shins**
3. **Hamstrings**
4. **Buttocks**
5. **Groin/inner thigh**
6. **Pelvic floor**

Tempo, Reps and Sets:

Tempo is the speed of the exercise. It is denoted by 4 numbers. The first number is the speed of lowering the weight. The second number is the pause at the bottom.

The third number is the speed of lifting the weight, pulling or pressing the weight or body. The last number is the pause at the top or the peak of the contraction.

Reps is short for repetitions or the number of times you repeat the exercise.

Sets denotes how many blocks of the given exercise you do. e.g. 2 sets of 10 reps or 3 sets of 8 reps.

A sample tempo for calves would be 2,1,1,1, you could do 8-12 reps and 3 sets.

I have just given samples here as there are multiple variables of sets and reps depending on the type of program you are doing. This is the science of program design. My goal here is simply to present exercises that will activate and train the muscles of the root chakra.

The Feet

The force generation sequence in the human body is from the ground up. Healthy feet are a critical component of overall healthy biomechanics. Foot problems are incredibly common among all age groups from fallen arches to inappropriate weight bearing patterns to a propensity to sprained ankles as a few examples. You cannot be properly anchored in your body without healthy feet.

There are movement schools like Yoga and Pilates that pay special attention to the feet. Many other exercise forms do not so I am going to include some exercises that will address this area. These exercises are good for prehab (preventing injury) and rehab (recovering from injury). They are all best done in bare feet.

Treading

This is an exercise that's normally done on a Pilates reformer but this modified version can be done standing on the floor or, even better, standing on a step to get extra range of motion. If you do it on a step you need to be able to hold onto something so a stairway would work well for home exercisers and a step in a squat rack for gym goers. The benefit of just doing it on the floor in an open space without holding on is that you will train your balance, which will exercise the small muscles in your feet more.

Stand in place feet about hip distance apart and lift one heel up as high as you can. Your knee bends. Now change position by lowering that heel to the floor and lifting the other one. Continue this alternating pattern of lifting and lowering the heels. If you are on the elevated step or stairs then place the ball of the foot on the step and let the heel hang over. This way you can lower the heel down deeper to get a nice stretch for the Achilles tendon/calf region.

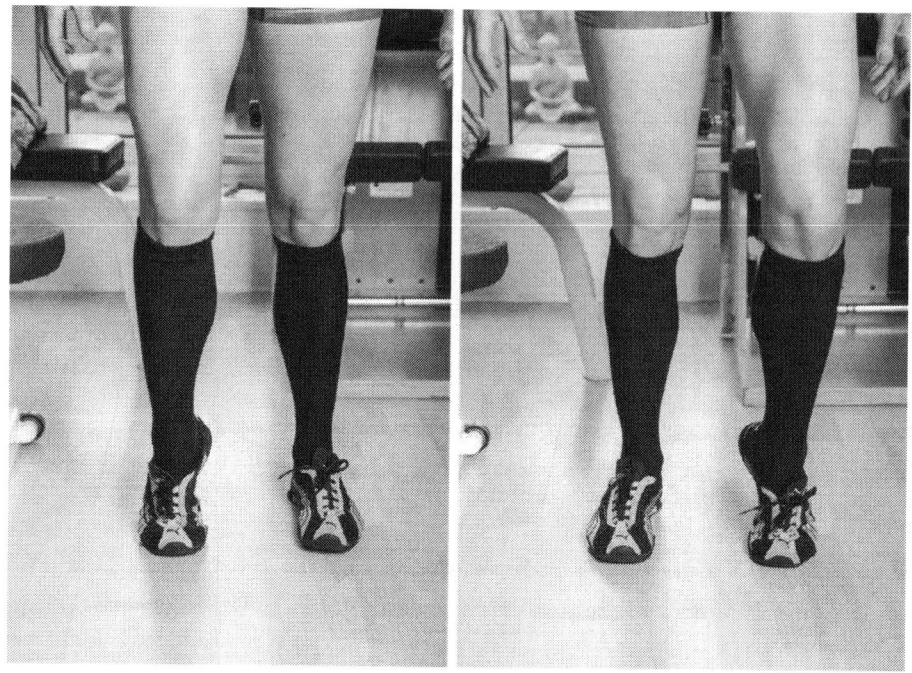

Treading

Walking series

Practice the following walking drills in bare feet to target the small muscles of the feet:

A. Walking only on the balls of the feet.

B. Walking only on the heels of the feet.

C. Walking on the inside edge of the feet.

D. Walking on outside edge of feet.

E. Walking using any of the above patterns on a dead straight line.

Each exercise can be done for distance or time about 30 seconds per exercise.

Foot balancing.

Again this is done bare foot. Stand tall, feet hip distance apart. Rise up onto the balls of both feet. Hold the balance for 30 to 60 seconds.

When you get good at the double leg you can do the single leg.

Simply rise up onto ball of one foot and keep other one off the ground. Hold the balance from 30 – 60 seconds.

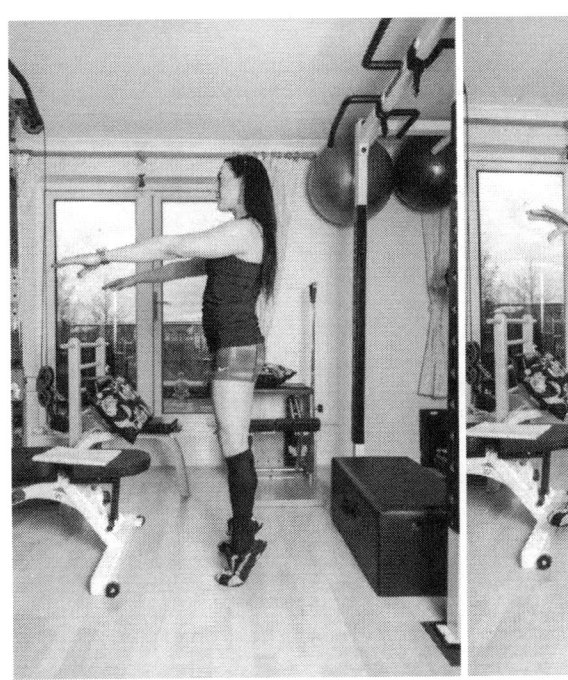

Foot Balancing on two feet

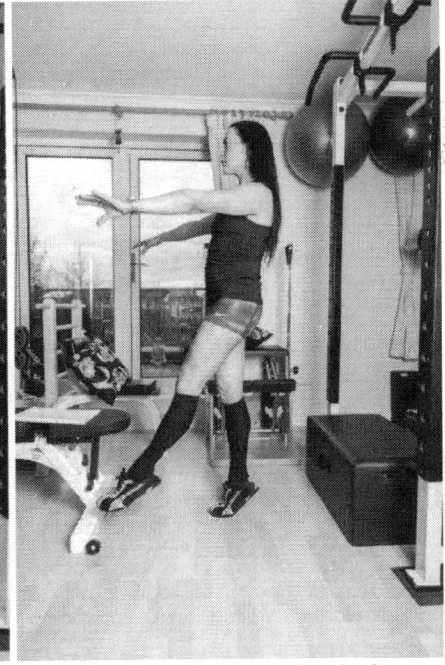

Foot Balancing one foot at a time

Calves and Shins

Smith Machine Calf Raise

Set yourself up in a smith machine with a step. Stand on the edge of the step, balls of the feet on and heels over the edge, bar of the machine on your back. The feet are pointing forward. Inhale as you lower the heels down over the edge of the step. Pause for a second at the bottom till you get a good stretch and press up while squeezing the calves.

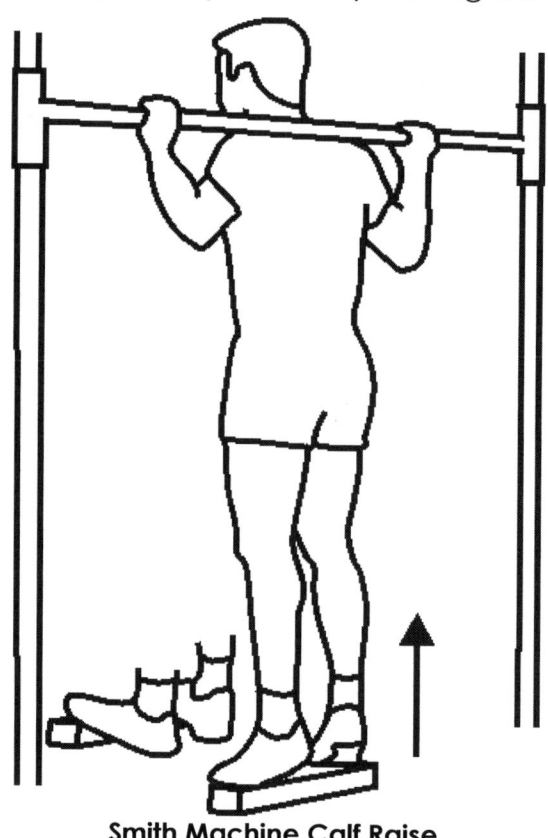

Smith Machine Calf Raise

Stairwell Calf raises Single Leg

This is a version of the above exercise that can be done at home. It's the very same as the one above only you stand on the bottom step of the stairs with one leg on the ball of your foot. You can increase the resistance by holding a dumbbell in one hand.

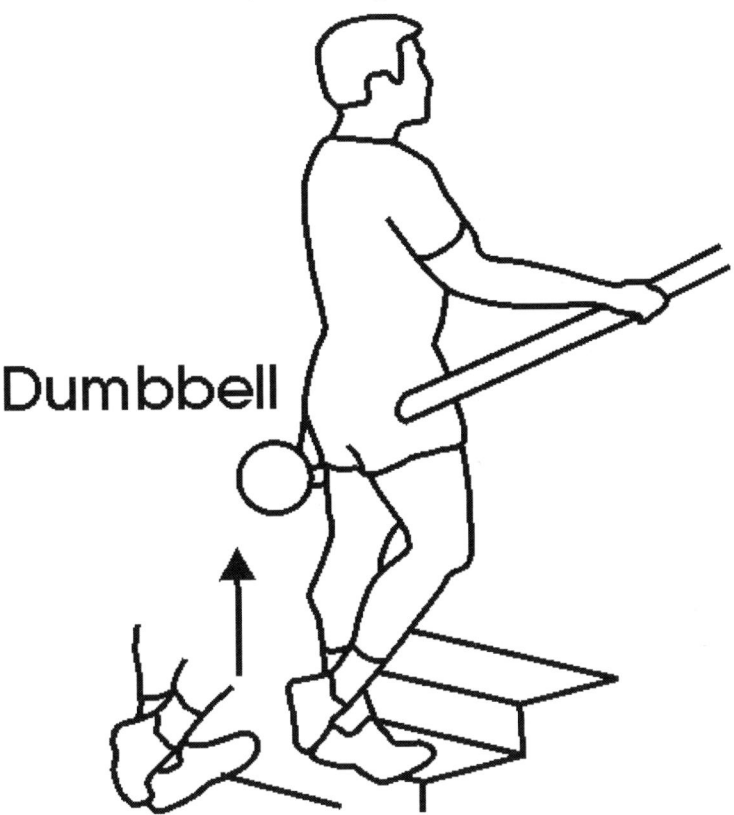

Toe press with Band.

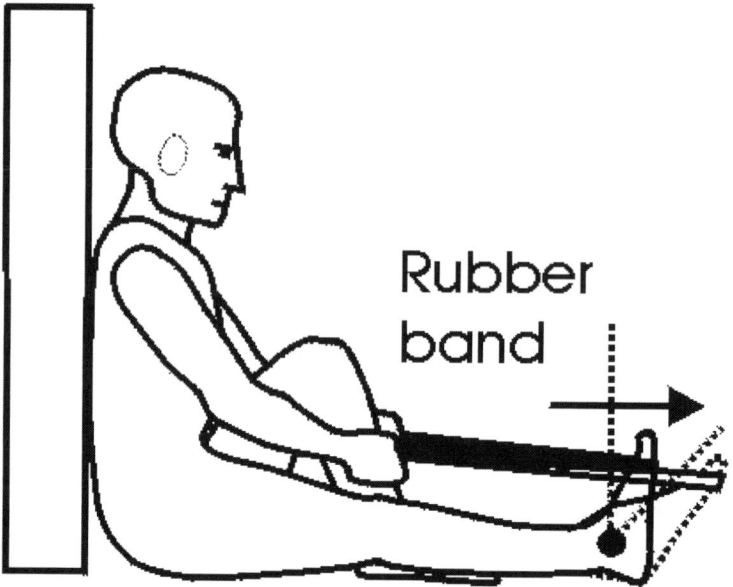

This one can be done seated or laying down on the back with the foot at right angles. Inhale to pull toe back towards the body then exhale to press the toe away from the body while squeezing the calf. If one side is weaker you can do it first.

Seated Calf Raise

This can be done in the gym or at home. Make sure there is a spongy collar or large towel wrapped around the bar. The bar is placed on upper thighs close to the knees. Feet are placed hip width apart with the balls of the feet on a step and the heels over the edge. Inhale as you lower the heels deep. Pause for a second and then exhale as you press up to a peak contraction in the muscles.

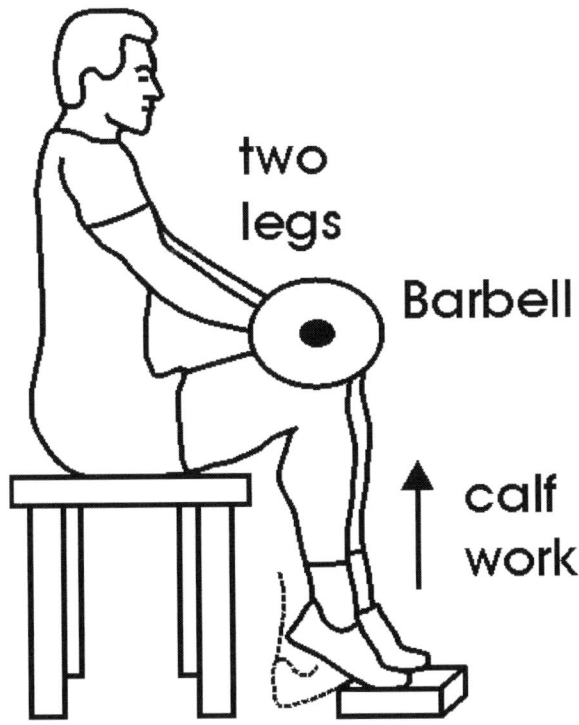

Plate raise

In order to have a balanced lower leg we need to train the muscles in the front. To target the muscles in the shins place a weight plate gently over one foot. Now try to lift the toes up toward the shins. You should feel a contraction in the front of the shins. (Sample tempo 2,0,1,1)

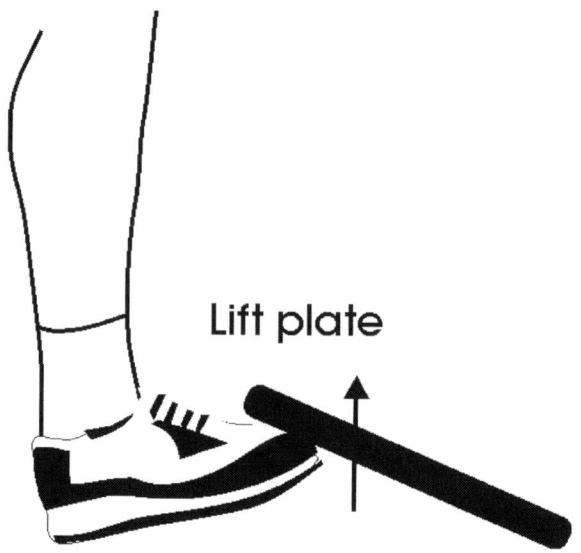

Tibialis pull

This exercise can be done in the gym at a cable station with a loop attachment or at home using a band that you attach to a table leg for example. Loop the band around your foot and sit tall. Pull the toes back towards the shin. Hold the contraction for a second and release back as you continue focus on the muscular tension. Sample tempo; 2,0,1,1

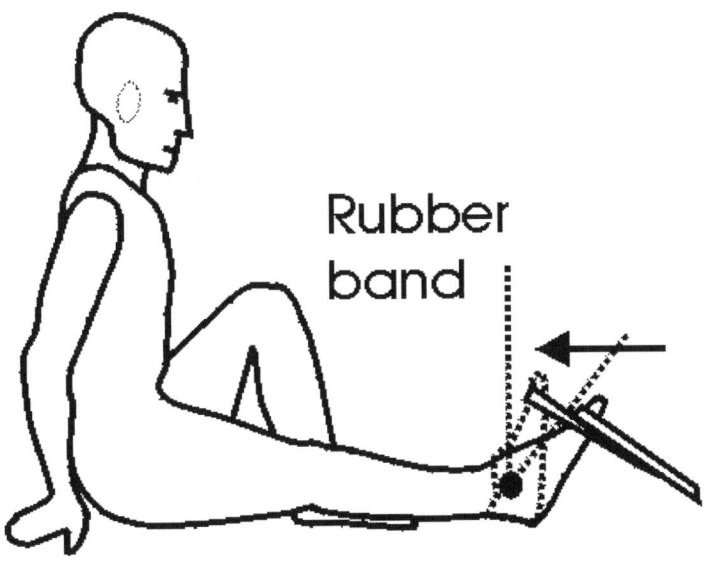

Hamstrings

Sample tempo for the hamstrings 4,0,1,0 , Sample reps 6-8, Sample sets 3

Hamstring Curl on the Ball

This is a great introductory exercise for the hamstrings or back of the thighs. It can also be done at home as you just need a Swiss ball. Get on your back and place your feet in a parallel position on a Swiss ball. Squeeze butt and lift hips up in the air. Freeze this position. Now pull the ball in towards your butt. Slowly move the ball back to the start position. You can do more reps than usual with this exercise as you can't progress it with load. You can go as high as 15-20 reps. If you are doing the higher reps reduce the tempo.

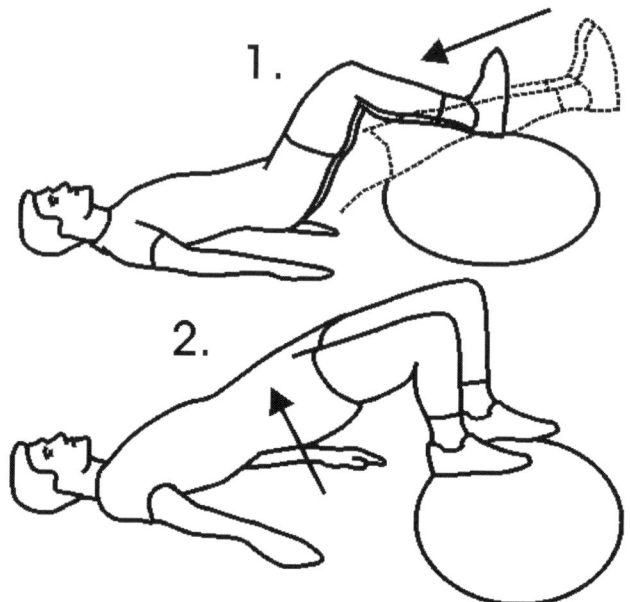

Hamstring Curl with Swiss ball

Prone hamstring curl

This exercise is done in the gym using a machine. Lay face down on the machine and hold on securely, feet hooked around pads. Keep your butt down at all times. Exhale to pull your heels towards your butt. Slowly lower with control to a full straightening of the legs. Full range of motion is an important principle for maximal recruitment of all of the muscle fibres.

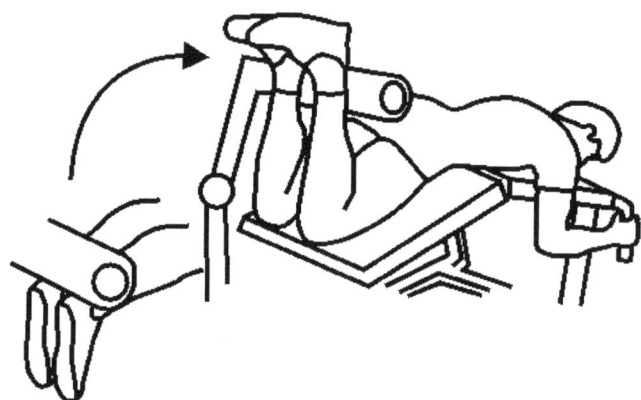

Prone hamstring curl

Supine Band Hamstring Arc

Lie on ground and wrap a band around base of foot, elbows glued to floor. Exhale to push the foot towards the floor and inhale as you bring it up to close to 90 degrees depending on flexibility. You can easily do up to 20 reps with this one with a slightly slower tempo of 3010. If you have a weaker side you do it first.

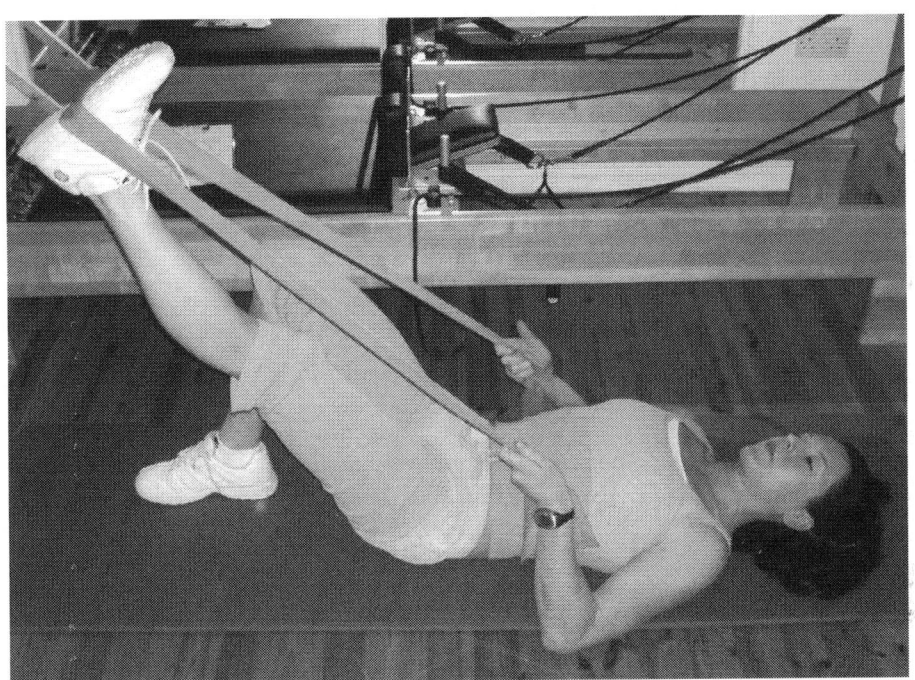

Supine Band Hamstring Arc

Standing Hamstring Curl using a Pulley

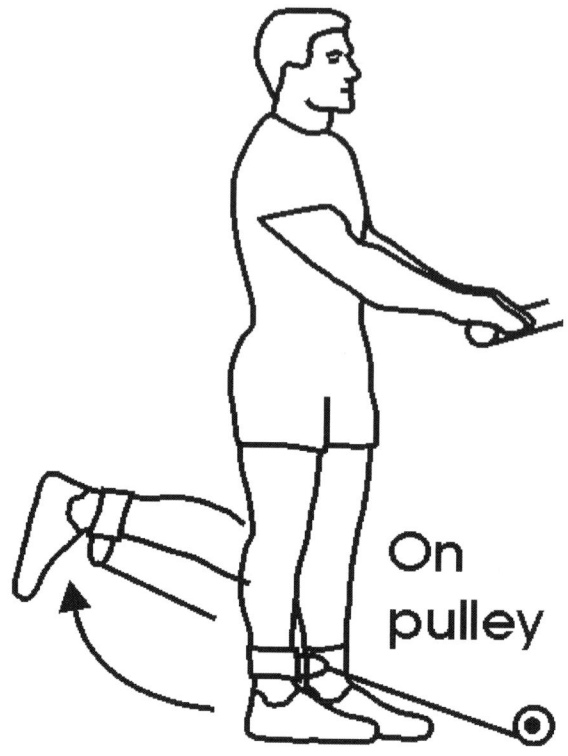

You need to work with a cable station at the gym for this one. Get the appropriate attachment to attach your foot to the cable connection. It's usually a strap that you put around your ankle. Start with the weaker side. Make sure there is a small bend in the knee to stabilise the standing leg. Exhale to pull the heel to the butt and inhale to slowly lower back to the start getting a full range of motion. Make sure you are also holding on securely to the cable station.

Single leg Hip lift

This exercise will target the hamstrings one at a time (It also hits the buttocks). It's handy as you can use it for a home program. Lay on your back close to a sturdy chair or bench. Organise yourself so that your thigh is at about 90 degrees and your heel is securely on the chair or bench. Press heel into chair, squeeze butt and lift hips right off the ground till knee, hip and shoulder are in a straight line. Slowly lower to the start position.

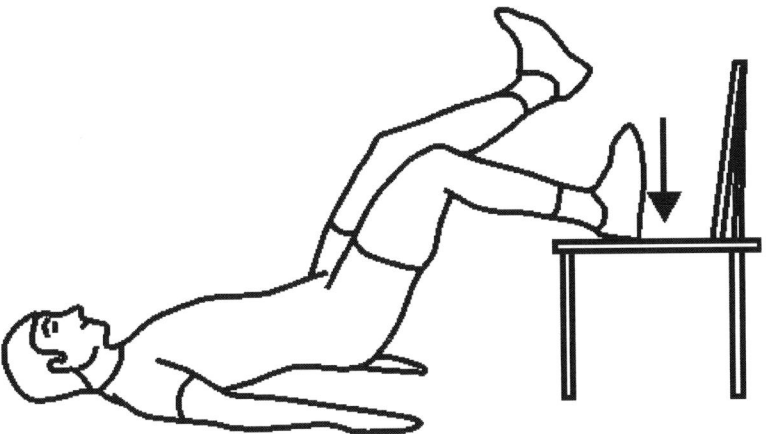

Buttocks

The buttocks are one of the most inhibited muscle groups in the whole of the human body. I have never come across a client that had great buttock function from the beginning. From a biomechanical perspective the reasons for this can be related to our limited range of motion about the hips.

Squatting down to a deep position like a baby does is not something that happens for most individuals past early childhood. From an energetic perspective I call the buttocks the "seat of power". If you are not fully in your power, and let's face it not many people are, this muscle group cannot really function properly.

The exercises that follow will start to biomechanically correct the functioning of the muscles and also energetically reawaken them. On many levels dis-ease and dysfunction are simply a blockage in the flow of energy. Exercising your muscles with real focus, sometimes called mind/body connection, exponentially generates a healing effect for your body and being.

Buttock Activator

When training a muscle group that's really inhibited and disconnected one of the most important things is to get the ball rolling again. We need to find an exercise that acts like a spark plug igniting the muscle group out of its sleepy state. The exercise I recommend as the starting point for the buttocks is the buttock squeeze.

If you have difficulty with this exercise it really shows the degree of inhibition that's present. Please however persist! Simply clench your butt cheeks together and relax them. Repeat this over and over. Aim to get to 20 reps initially and build it up to 50 in a given practice period. Squeeze, relax, squeeze and relax! Practice by standing with knees slightly bent. Practice seated. Practice lying on your tummy. Squeeze, relax, squeeze, and relax! You can place your hands on your buttocks while practicing to enhance the mind body connection. Get squeezing!

Hip lift on the Ball.

Sit on your exercise ball (also known as a Swiss ball) and walk out carefully until you are on your back. Your shoulders should be on the apex of the ball and your head parallel to the ceiling. Place your hands on your hips and align your feet in a "V" position as opposed to parallel. Inhale as you lower your butt to the floor. Now exhale and press straight back up. Give the buttocks an extra squeeze at the top for 1 to 2 seconds. You can progress the exercise by holding a medicine ball at hips or a barbell. Make sure you are using an anti-burst ball for safety. Sample tempo for buttock exercises: 3, 0 ,1,1

-Barbell
-Hip raise

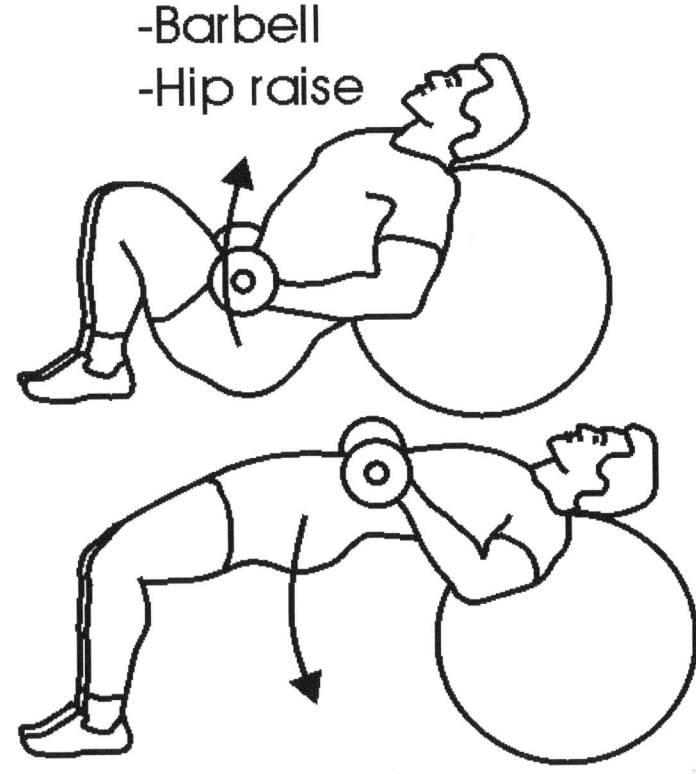

Reverse Hyper

Once again you can use the Swiss ball here. In the gym as a progression you can use a reverse hyper machine if it's available. Lay tummy down on the ball with hands on the floor. Start with legs in a "V" position, spread apart. Now lift up the legs by really squeezing the buttocks. At the same time bring the feet together. Give an extra hard squeeze of the buttocks before lowering to the "V" position again.

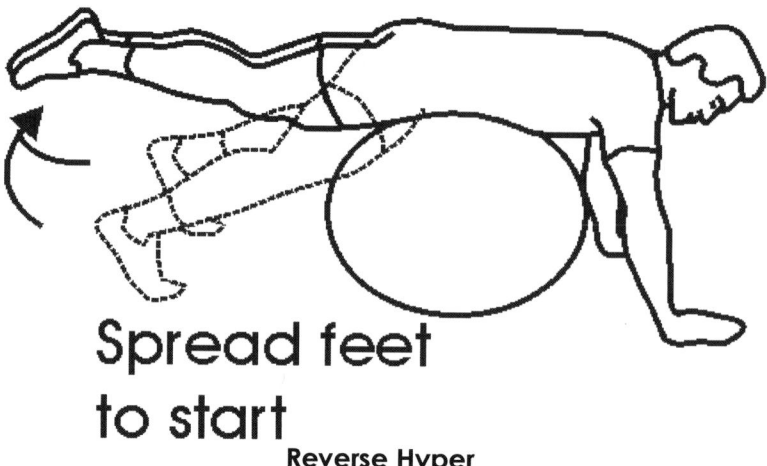

Spread feet to start

Reverse Hyper

Box Squat

This is a move that has been used by power-lifters for decades. It can also be used by beginners to start the process of activating the buttocks. Use a bench or box that is secure. Stand in front of it but close to it with feet well outside of the hips with toes turned out about 25 degrees. Inhale as you lower your butt down onto the bench maintaining a neutral spine. You can reach your hands forward to assist your balance as you learn this move. Later to progress you can hold a medicine ball or weight plate at your waist. Advanced trainees will work using a loaded barbell on the upper traps. In every case but especially the higher the load you use be sure to never bounce off the bench. Keep constant tension on the buttocks and neutral spine throughout. I never recommend less than 6-8 reps in this exercise.

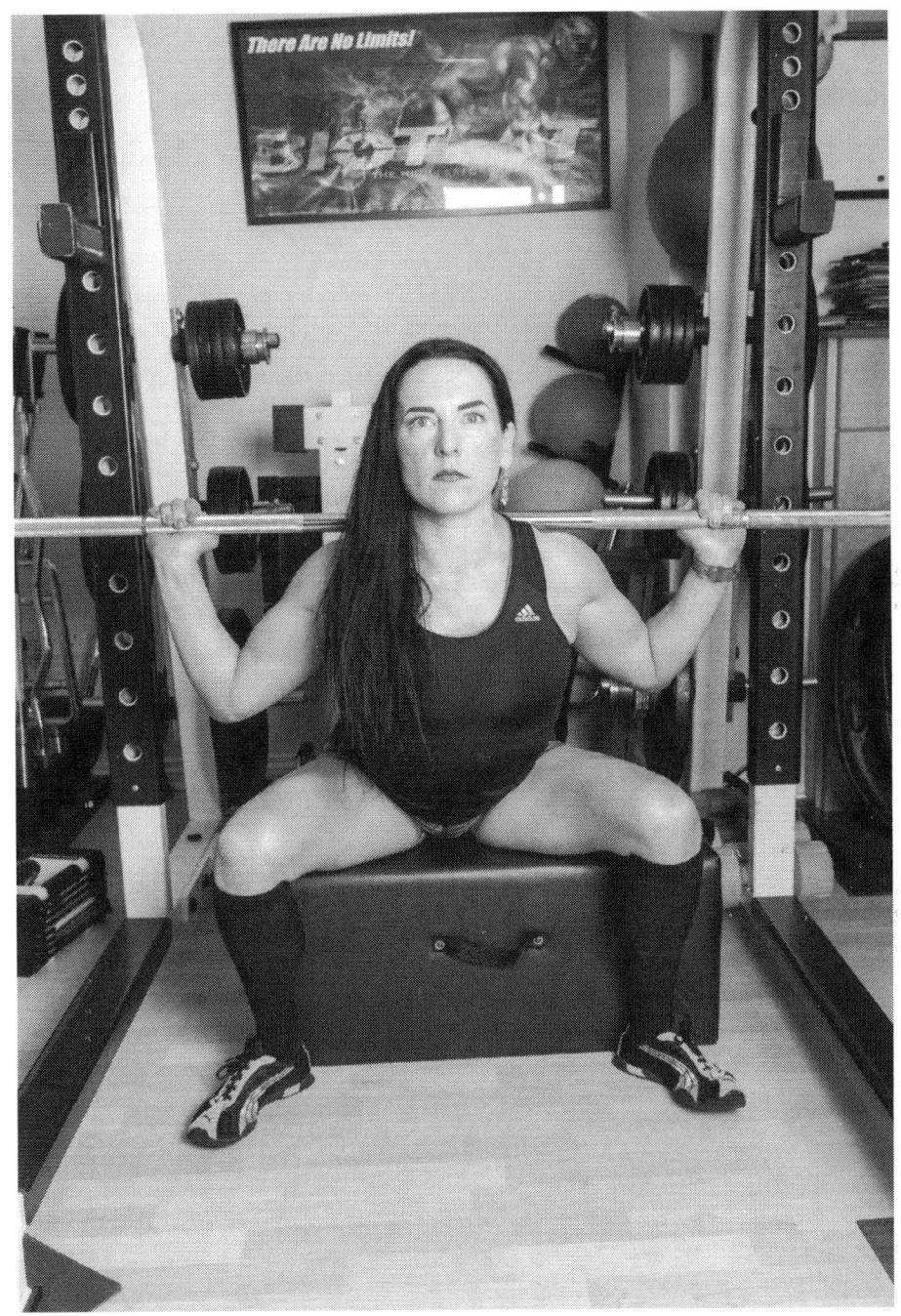

Box Squat

Back Squat

This is an exercise that has to be prepared for with the appropriate stretches so that one can achieve the best range which is as deep as possible. In strength training circles it's known as "ass to the grass"!

Beginners can start with body weight reaching the hands forward as a counterbalance. For many people elevating the heels on to weight plates can really help achieve a better depth of squat. Try 2 x 5kg plates to start. Just place the heels on the plates with the balls of the feet on the floor toes turned out 15 degrees.

Begin the squat by imagining you are in double glazing. Put your knees through the double glazing and immediately descend with the trunk keeping a neutral spine, chest up and eyes level with the horizon. Drive up with a strong buttock squeeze to the start. Keep your elbows directly under the bar.

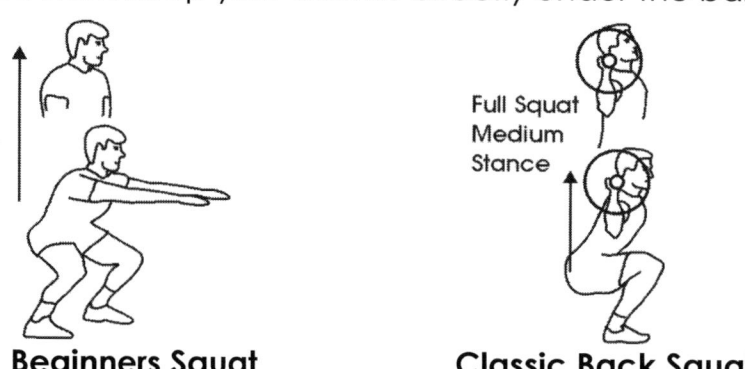

Beginners Squat **Classic Back Squat**

GROIN /INNER THIGH

When testing many of my clients I see a lot of bilateral adductor weakness. This means the muscles of the groin are really shut down. This is a sign of adrenal fatigue which is incredibly common in today's modern world of relentless stress. The first exercise is a gentle introduction to getting the energy flowing here again. Sample tempo 3,0,1,0. Sample reps 12-15. Sample sets, 3.

Open/Close

Lay on your back with arms either resting by side or tucked in under the buttocks. Raise legs up as high as you can to get close to 90 degrees without losing neutral spine (neutral spine is when you can lay on your back and slip your hand in the gap of the lower back and maintain this space throughout the exercise). Inhale as you open the legs as wide as possible. Maintain a conscious engagement of your pelvic floor by squeezing the muscles that control bladder and bowel. Now exhale to bring the legs back together again as you concentrate on using the muscles of the inner thighs. This exercise can be progressed by wrapping and exercise band around each foot and pinning your elbows to the floor. Continue the leg movement in and out against the resistance.

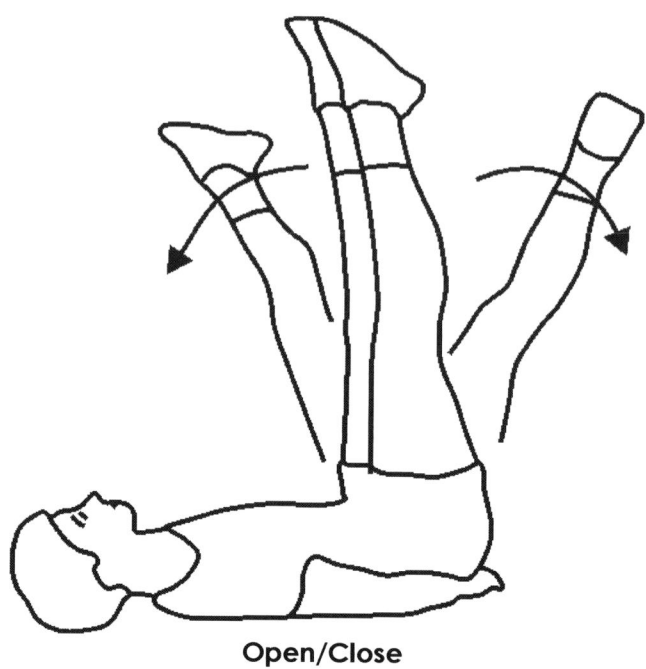

Open/Close

Ball squeeze

Lay on the back with the ball between the knees. If it's a big ball the ball can rest on the floor. Inhale first, and then as you exhale squeeze the ball together for 6 seconds at about 50 % effort. Repeat 6-8 times.

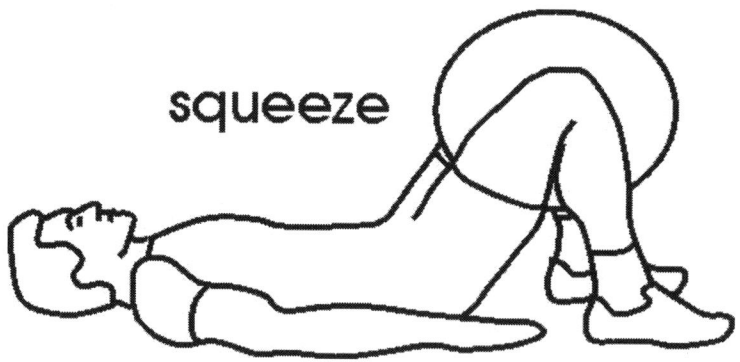

Adductor Machine Press

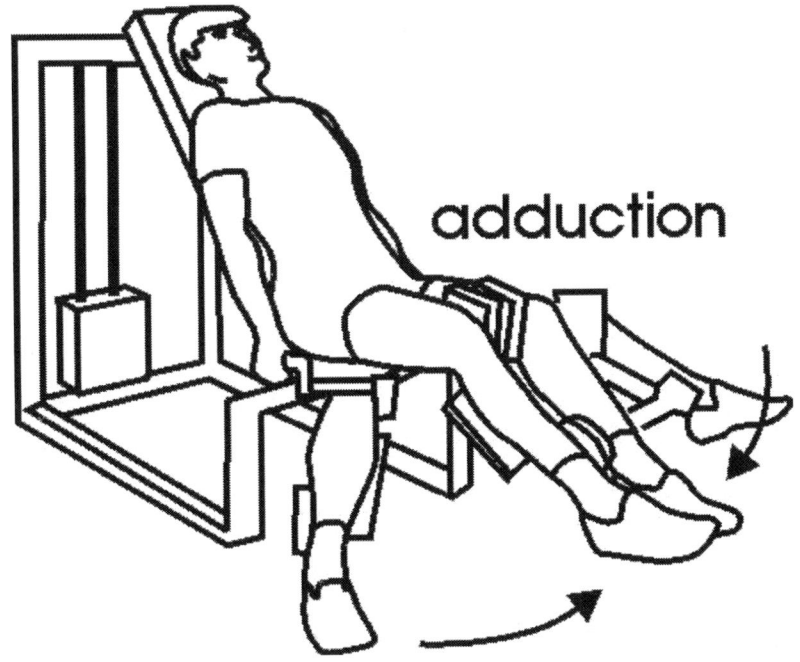

This exercise is done at a gym with one of these machines. Sit onto the machine with legs on the pads. Breathe in. As you exhale squeeze legs together while focusing on the inner thighs (adductors). Inhale to open the legs as wide as the machine and your body will allow.

Split Squat

This is another exercise I learned from Charles Poliquin. It is an exercise that really delivers on so many levels! One of those levels is a retraining of the muscles of the groin. One needs a minimum standard of flexibility in the hip although persisting with the exercise itself will also really help with flexibility. Place one foot on a low step or platform with foot turned out 15 degrees, chest up, rear foot facing forward and weight on the ball of the rear foot. Inhale as you lunge forward all the way until the thigh touches the calf. Really focus on keeping the trunk upright. It helps for some people to focus on leaning back. Go so far into the movement that the knee passes the toe. Exhale to press back up again. Really keep your pelvic floor engaged by squeezing the muscles that control bladder and bowel. If your inner thighs are weak you will particularly feel the effects of this the next day if it's your first time to do it.

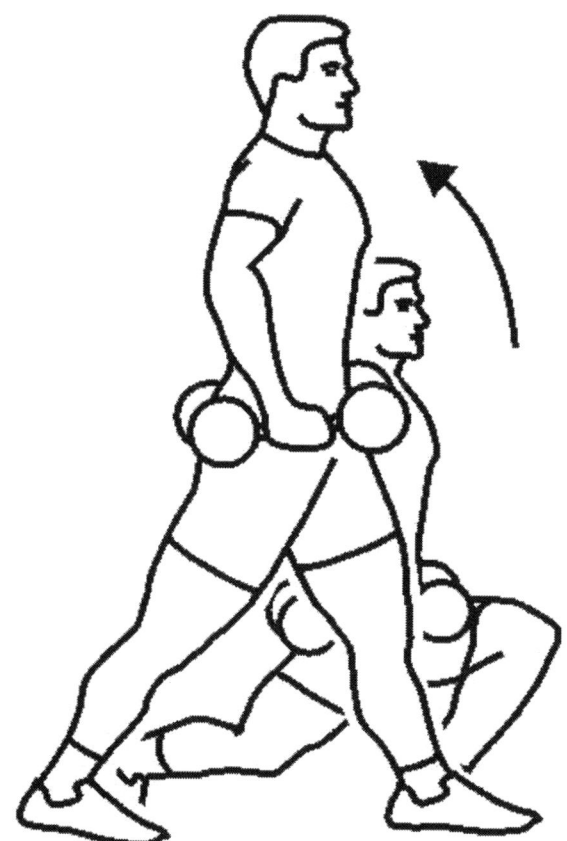

Split Squat: Front foot may be elevated on a step for ease of range

Walking Lunge

This exercise looks easy but for a beginner that may have flexibility, stability and co-ordination issues it is very demanding! One should master the split squat before introducing this more dynamic sister exercise. Start with your body weight and give yourself a decent amount of space to do your steps. Start with a big step forward going down nice and deep till your hamstring covers your calf. Keep your trunk nice and upright. Drive back up to two feet side by side position. Now take the next step forward with the opposite leg. Continue for anything from 12 to 24 steps. Progress the exercise by holding dumbbells in each hand.

When you do this exercise correctly you can feel how the inner thighs have been really well stimulated. You usually notice this about 24 – 48 hours after the workout.

Walk forward

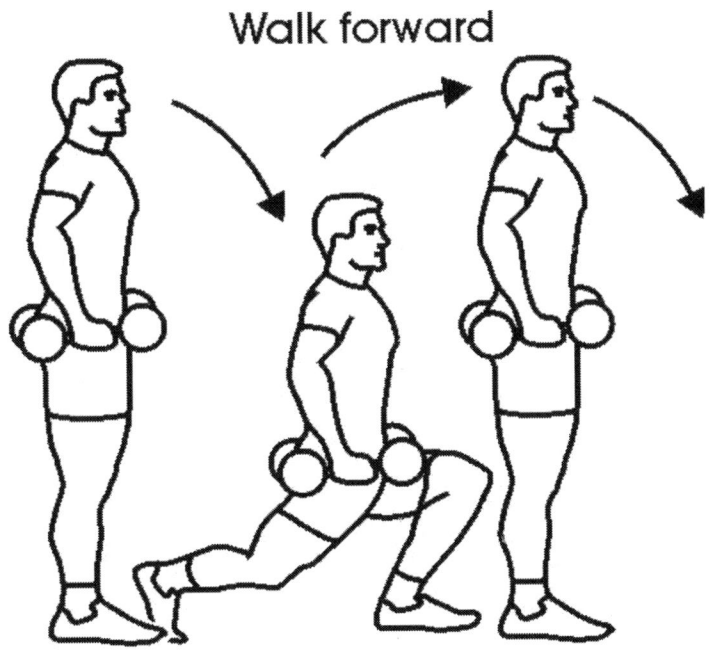

Pelvic Floor

The Pelvic Floor is a series of muscles around your groin area. If you are able to consciously feel the muscles that control your bladder and your bowel you have a mind/body connection to the pelvic floor. By squeezing the sphincter muscle that controls the bladder and simultaneously squeezing the sphincter muscle of the "back passage" there will be a global recruitment of all the pelvic floor musculature. If you are unsure simply try starting and stopping the "flow" the next time you use the toilet. Once you can do this the mind/body connection is established. You can practice these exercises practically anywhere.

On/Off

Zip up your pelvic floor by engaging the muscles that control bladder and bowel. Shoot for 50% effort (estimate this). Now relax completely. Zip it up again and relax again. Start the zip up and stop it on and off for 60 seconds.

The Elevator

Imagine you are in a building with an elevator. "0" on the elevator represents the ground floor or no pelvic floor function (incontinence). Floor 1 and 2 represent the residual tension that is always present in the pelvic floor that prevents incontinence and holds all of your internal organs in place. Now take a breath in. On the exhale zip up the pelvic floor a notch to an imagined 3rd floor. Hold this tension here, breath in and on the exhale take the zip up higher to level 5 (50% of a potential maximum). Hold this tension again and breathe in. This time on the exhale go up to level 7. Hold. Breathe and take it up to 9 and finally one last effort up to level 10 for an all-out max. Relax down to the residual tension that's always there.

Traffic Light Stop.

This time engage your zip up to 50 % effort and hold for 60 seconds. I call this one the traffic light as you can practice it in the car at a traffic light (or anywhere else it suits you!).

Chapter 7

Stress: Dealing with the "Fight/ Flight or Freeze Response."

The root chakra is the seat of the fight or flight response. Have you ever heard the expression "frightened out of the seat of your pants?" Well that is a root chakra phenomenon and not a great one if it's relentless. Now, getting the odd fright could" save your ass" in an emergency situation, like jumping out of the way of a car speeding toward you. Getting a bit of an adrenaline pump before attempting a maximal lift is most likely essential if you are going to be successful in that attempt. But the daily grind of stressors, traffic, deadlines, arguments with spouses, conflicts with co-workers and skipped meals to mention but a few all add up to the modern man and woman being in a state of hyper arousal or constant adrenaline pump. Stress is multi-faceted and all pervasive in the modern world. It is totally at odds with being in the body! You cannot be present if you are "frightened out of the seat of your pants".

So what can we do to deal with this fight/ flight or freeze response? There are many techniques that you will find helpful. They can be used separately or collectively to pack a more powerful punch.

Exercise

Exercise has been shown time and time again to be very beneficial for multiple markers of health. Indeed the health of our root chakra is possibly the most potent predictor of our overall health, vitality and most likely even our lifespan. The root chakra represents not only vitality and energy but also the will to live.

The root chakra governs the physical structure of our body's' muscle, bone and connective tissue. These tissues collectively (with internal organs) constitute a phenomenon called lean body mass. Your lean body mass is the tissue that remains once the fat has been subtracted from the equation.

Research from Tufts University shows us that our number one predictor of lifespan is how much lean body mass we maintain over the course of a lifetime. Sarcopenia is an age related disease of muscle wasting. The word comes from Greek meaning poverty of flesh. In modern science it's called muscle atrophy.

The second predictor of lifespan is how strong a person is. We can see factor 1 and 2 on the hit list of longevity are intricately entwined. Without a sufficient amount of muscle it's difficult to be strong. Without training for strength, muscle mass cannot easily be maintained or developed further. It is with this rationale that I see that weightlifting is the greatest contributor to root chakra health. Weight training stimulates muscle mass development and strength development way above and beyond any other form of training.

Weight training in a progressive and planned form offers endless variety. It is the single best modality to maintain bone density. With correct guidance a novice can train safely.

Those who have hormonal disturbances can also benefit from specialised program design to offset the issues in question. Take, for example, adrenal fatigue (the result of a constant and over stimulation of the adrenal glands in a variety of stress responses) as an issue that can be helped with weight training. If one lifts intensely with heavier weight and less reps (around the 6-8 rep mark is ideal for beginners, experienced lifters can go heavier) and has longer rest intervals (about 3 minutes on average) this is a lot kinder to the adrenals than long distance running or other forms of endurance exercise.

Using the Chinese system of Yin and Yang, exercise can be classed as Yin style or Yang style. Weight lifting is a Yang style of training. One needs to be careful with Yang style exercise if your root chakra is massively depleted. Remember your root chakra can be blocked, hyperactive or depleted. If it's very depleted a Yin style of exercise would be ideal to build up a minimum baseline amount of chi or energy. A classic example of this would be doing the root chakra energy exercises in this book. When one is healthier the Yin exercises can complement the Yang style training and help one recover to best effect.

Yin is the "oil" and Yang is the "fire" or outward expression of power. Without the oil we can have no fire. When the oil runs low we need to replenish it. Other examples of Yin exercises include certain styles of Yoga (the gentler slower moving styles rather than the more aggressive dynamic styles), Pilates, Tai Chi and Qigong.

Training your Legs as a Base Chakra must.

"Be sure to put your feet in the right place, then stand firm."
Abraham Lincoln

Our bodies, perhaps more than any other aspect of ourselves, are one of our greatest tools for self- awareness and self- development. Reason being- the body never lies! You can lie to yourself, you can lie to your spouse , you can lie to your friends and family but your body, that ever faithful friend will always tell you the truth .The body tells us this truth , not in words but in feelings, sensations, perceptions and simply by how it looks , moves and performs.

How your legs look, how strong they are, how symmetrical they are, how structurally balanced they are speaks volumes about the individual.

In the upright environment, standing on your two feet moving around or participating in sports, forces are generated from the ground up. Studies of elite boxers show that over 70% of the power of the punch is generated from the legs. Novice Olympic lifters and field sport athletes (shot, hammer etc.) start out developing 80 % of the power for lifting the weight or throwing the implement from their upper bodies. Ten years of training later the elite experienced lifter/field athlete now generates 80% of the power from the legs with the upper body contributing only 20% of the power. In my estimation athleticism is mostly about learning how to use your legs to the greatest potential.

Mastery of the physical plane if you are a human being will always be enhanced by getting your legs strong especially in that upright setting. So if your training program does not include plenty of squats and deadlifts with auxiliary exercises, like split squats and deadlift variations your legs will not be well served nor will your entire life experience. You see your legs are governed by your root and sacral chakras(chakra 2) respectively.

Your root chakra connects you to the earth. The theme of this chakra is safety, security, survival, and tribal issues (in the modern world this means family, in the scientific world this means genetics.)

The root chakra is the chakra of NOW! Those who are living in the now will have a strong root chakra. There is nothing like some heavy squatting or deadlifting to bring you exquisitely into the now. Being in the now is the ultimate security. All fear, for the most part, comes from worrying about what might happen in the future.

In bodybuilding circles many believe that good legs are simply genetic. Well if you have good genes (a root chakra phenomenon) then you may have a head start. In order to get the best legs for aesthetics or performance you have to do "the leg work". For this reason the strength and functioning of the legs are in many ways reflective of the individuals' work ethic, discipline and mental toughness.

Skinny weak legs equal a weak root chakra. The root chakra is the chakra of manifestation. So if you are not realising your goals and dreams, maybe you should be squatting more!

Legs covered in a deep layer of fat represent emotional suppression and or a traumatic childhood. The energetics of the first two chakras develop in the early childhood years. In western science we call it Oestrogen Dominance. Show me a person with severe Oestrogen Dominance who is not an emotional basket case (at least once a month!).

Legs that are skinny are reflective of the overall muscle mass of the body. It's rare to see someone with impressive leg development without overall body development. The opposite cannot be said.

Participants in a study called the Danish MONICA project reported in the British Medical journal September 2009 came to the following conclusion:

"A low thigh circumference seems to be associated with an increased risk of developing heart disease or premature death. The adverse effects of small thighs might be related to too little muscle mass in the region. The measure of thigh circumference might be a relevant anthropometric measure to help general practitioners in early identification of individuals at an increased risk of premature morbidity and mortality." [1]

Your legs are a metaphor for so many things:

- Standing up for yourself (self-respect)
- Holding your ground
- Standing strong
- Standing for what you believe in
- Doing the Leg work
- Taking steps to achieve something

If you are a guy and you like lean legs in a woman maybe you are subconsciously looking for someone who is emotionally evolved.

If you are a female and you like a man with strong well developed legs maybe you are attracted to the good genetics or work ethic they may represent! Whatever way you slice it strong lean legs are a platform for a grander life experience.

Meditation

Meditation has been recommended by most spiritual gurus as a path to freedom and enlightenment. Even if your goals are more practical than Spiritual it can serve you well as a stress reduction tool. All stress creates one of two things 1) a monkey mind of constant crazy thinking 2) a raft of lower harmonic emotions (anger, rage, frustration, blame, guilt etc.). The direction that meditation aims to guide the individual toward is a state of pure "Being".

A state of pure consciousness/awareness that is devoid of thought and free of the lower harmonics of emotion. In this state a person experiences at a minimum a state of peace and tranquillity and for more practiced subjects a state of exhilaration or bliss.

When thought and feeling/emotions stop, awareness begins. Thoughts and emotions are like a layer of crap that covers up our inner radiance. This radiance is brimming over with joy. How do we get to this most apparently elusive state? There are many roads but one of the tried and trusted methods is meditation. Meditation can be done in stillness or it can be done with movement.

Meditation for the root chakra:

Stand with the feet just outside hip distance apart with toes turned out about 45 degrees. Place hands, palms facing the body, just in front of the lower abdominal wall in between the pubic bone and belly button. This region is sometimes referred to as the "soul seat" (also known as the lower Dan Tien).

1: Now visualise yourself standing on a big globe representing the earth.

2: Imagine this earth globe is sliced in half and you can see right through to the molten core of the earth.

3: Imagine you are standing on a grassy bank or muddy one or sand. Ideally you practice this in bare feet to maximise the feeling of contact with the ground (Mother Earth).

4: Next imagine a red beam of light coming out from your pelvic floor going down and penetrating the earth.

Imagine it traveling deeper and deeper till it merges with the molten core of the earth.

5: Now to start the movement. Breath in to prepare. Exhale as you lower into a ¼ squat position weight nicely distributed on the base of heels , base of the big toes and base of the little toes.

6: Inhale as you straighten to the start position. Visualise the red light constantly pulsing up and down.

7: As you lower downwards imagine gifting energy to the earth. As you come to the most upright position imagine receiving energy from the Earth.

Vitality Builder: The chi stick meditation

I learned this exercise many years ago from Paul Chek. It comes from the Qigong tradition. It is a very powerful exercise to cultivate chi or energy.

Stand with one foot in front of another in a martial arts stance. Make sure the knees are bent a little. Let your weight sink into your feet. Keep your chest up and spine neutral. Hold a small stick or ruler (about 12 inches long) inbetween the palms of the hands (direct connection to the heart chakra).

Reach out infront of you and make anticlockwise circles away from your body and back to it again. Decide on a certain number of repititions from 20 to 100 off each leg. Go nice and slow synchronising the breath in a continuous loop with the movement. Place the tongue on the roof of the mouth just behind the teeth.

This creates a connection between the principal front and back meridians of the body. Breathe in through the nose and out through the mouth. The bigger the circles the more energy one generates. The slower the movement the more energy or chi one generates. In the words of Moshe Feldenkrais, movement expert:

"The slower you go, the faster you get results!"

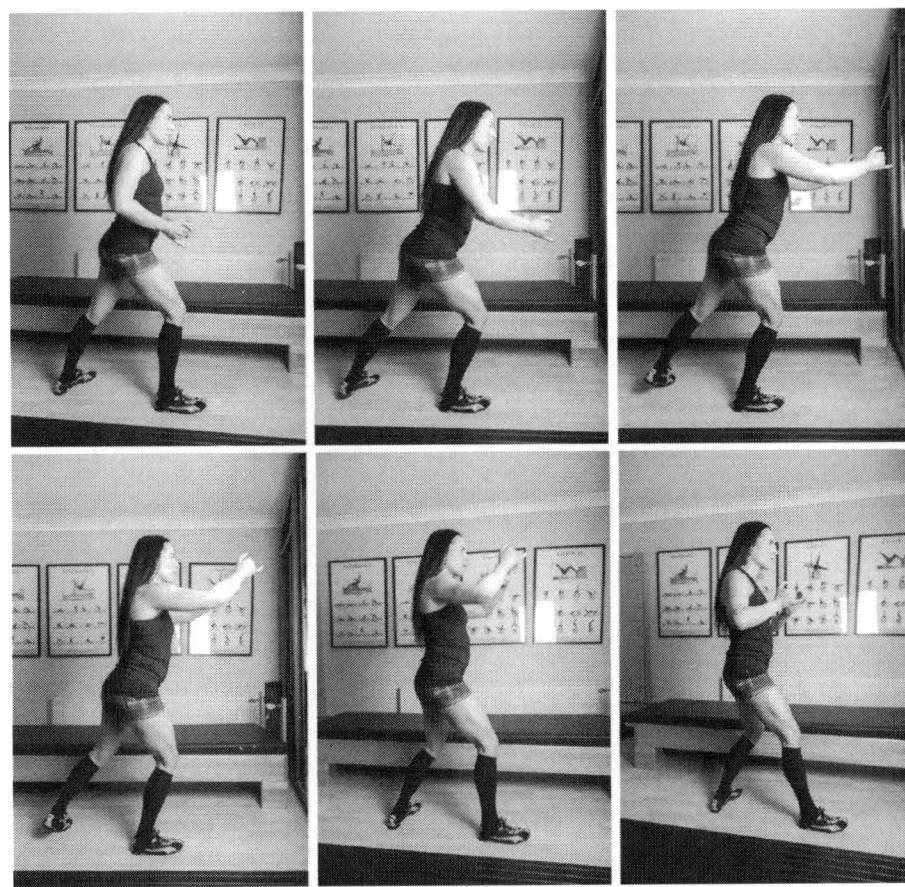

Chi Stick Moving Meditation

Nature Walks:

Going out in nature for a walk that is not "fitness" oriented, like a power walk, can be very regenerating for the root chakra. Your feet are connecting to the earth and your senses can be attuned to all that Mother Nature has to offer. Feel the ground beneath your feet.

Note the changes of terrain, the softness of the muddy banks, the firmness of a structured road, the uneven rocky terrain of an off raod track. Feel the sunlight on your skin or the breeze. Receive it in the moment. Notice it. Its like a communion with Mother Nature.

Walking Meditation:

When I go for a nature walk this is one of my favourite practices and its even better if you can do it barefoot, even if just for sections of your walk. Before you begin the walk do the following preparations.

Drop all of your barriers . You can just visualise walls dropping all around you.

Expand your energy body out. Just visualise a layer of light or multicoloured lights expanding out into infinity all around you.

Imagine taking plugs or stoppers out of the soles of your feet.

As you progress through your walk:

Ask your body now to dump or release through the soles of your feet everything that no longer serves you; toxic thoughts, toxic feelings, chemical toxins in the body, electromagnetic charge that you have accumulated, heaviness and /or contraction. Gift it to Gaia (Mother Earth) . She is a master recycler and loves to receive this energy!

As you walk ask the air, the earth, the grass, the ocean or any body of water, the birds and animals and trees to gift their healing energy to you. You gift to these elements in return by being aware of them, admiring their beauty and innocence and being grateful for them.

As you do your walk ask your body to relax more and more. Ask it to sink deeper and deeper into the earth

Gardening:

Digging the earth, feeling it with your hands, planting seeds, potting plants and planning the layout of your garden can all be ways of supporting your root chakra. Even growing a few herbs or tomato plants on your balcony can be a contribution for you. Fresh flowers in your home can also be an example of how Mother Nature can gift energy to you and your root chakra.

Pets:

Many studies show that pet owners enjoy better levels of health compared to those who do not have a pet. They have a calming effect reducing stress levels. Petting them, playing with them or simply hanging out with them increases serotonin levels. People with pets are shown to have lower levels of blood pressure, lesser incidence of cardiovascular disease and speedier recovery from a cardiac arrest if it does happen. Pets have often been prescribed for people suffering from depression. Having a dog for example encourages people to exercise with the daily walk. Pets show us how to live in the moment and love unconditionally.

Scientists at the Azuba University in Japan, have shown in their research that playing with your dog for 30 minutes while making eye contact increases oxytocin (a hormone in the human body connected with bonding and affection) by 20% [2]. Studies show that oxytocin acts to counteract the effects of the stress hormone cortisol[3].

Earthing/Grounding

The phenomenon of earthing/grounding has become more popular in recent years as many people are becoming more aware of the disturbance that living in an electromagnetic storm on a daily basis creates.

Human beings are electromagnetic entities. When our physical bodies are constantly bombarded by use of electrical devices and computers our own subtle electromagnetic balance becomes disturbed.

One of the simplest ways to off-set this disturbance is to walk outside barefoot or to swim in the sea or a mineral rich lake. This allows excess charge to dissipate and bring the body back to a state of electromagnetic harmony.

One study has shown that grounding has an effect on blood viscosity which reduces cardiovascular risk[4]. Another study on grounding indicated an effect on many physiological markers pertaining to health such as mineral status, blood sugar regulation and levels of thyroid hormones [5].

The awareness of this grounding phenomenon can be integrated into your life in many ways. You can walk outside barefoot, weather and conditions permitting, whenever possible. You can do your root chakra breathing squat meditation outside barefoot. You can swim in the sea or mineral rich lake. You can even purchase products to recreate a grounding effect like grounding sheets and mats that simulate the same effect as being outside barefoot.

Check out:

www.groundology.com

www.earthing.com

www.earthinginstitute.net

Chapter 8

Mindfulness with Movement

Bioenergy is the life force that animates, permeates and radiates from all things. Some cultures call it prana or chi. The ancient Yogis identified energy centres in the human body where this energy concentrates itself. These energy centres are classically defined as 7 chakras although many additional chakras and minor chakras have also been identified.

In western medicine these chakras seem to correspond to nerves plexuses (a network of intersecting nerves) and endocrine(hormone producing) organs. For the root chakra the nerve plexus is the sacral plexus and the endocrine glands are the adrenals and the testes.

Based on the last few chapters we see that we can modulate the energy and function of the chakras by things like nutrition therapy and exercise of the muscle groups pertaining to the chakra. We can also modulate the energy with a moving meditation. I like to call it mindful movement.

This is what the exercises that follow are. They are moving meditations to focus attention on the root chakra. I first learned this technique from Yoga and later in my work with Paul Chek.

Energy has its own intelligence and can unplug blockages, calm down hyperactivity, or stimulate greater activity depending on what the chakra requires.

Chakra energy can exist in 4 states; balanced, hyperactive, underactive and blocked. When all chakras are balanced we have energy, vitality and health. We are mentally physically emotionally and spiritually in a state of harmony and ease.

Simply by moving and focusing on the chakra with attentiveness the energy can come back to a state of balance if it was out of balance. The breathing should be deep and rhythmic allowing the belly to expand. The exercises should be practiced with regularity, ideally daily. A time frame of 10 minutes would be a nice starting point.

One can do a series of exercises for a given chakra or just one that feels the best for the duration of time chosen. Often times I like to close my eyes for bioenergy exercises so that my awareness can be more internalised and there is less chance of distraction. This is not always possible as some exercises are more desirable done with eyes open to assist balance.

Breathing Squat

Start in a standing position, feet just outside of hip width with the toes turned out. Place the palms out in front of you facing the body just above the pubic bone. This area corresponds to the centre of gravity, chakra 2 or lower Dan tien in Chinese medicine. It is the place where vital energy is stored and cultivated for use by the rest of the body. In this exercise it is like we are topping up this storage point via building the energy of the root chakra.

Keep the trunk nice and upright with a neutral spine. Neutral spine will have you with a small inward curvature of the lower back, a fully lifted chest, shoulders back and head resting nicely on the trunk with no forward protrusion. Now breath in to prepare, exhale as you bend the knees about ¼ squat depth (you can go deeper if you wish but I find it easier to pulse the energy slowly over a longer period of time without any fatigue or strain). Inhale to go back to the start position without locking out the knees. Continue up and down like that with a focus on exhale down, inhale up. Also keep focus on the pelvic floor.

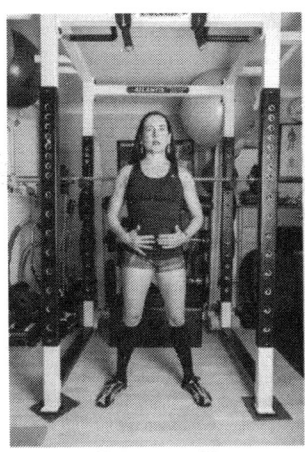 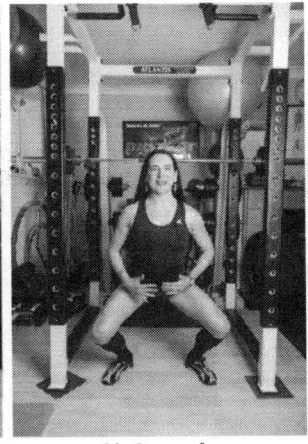 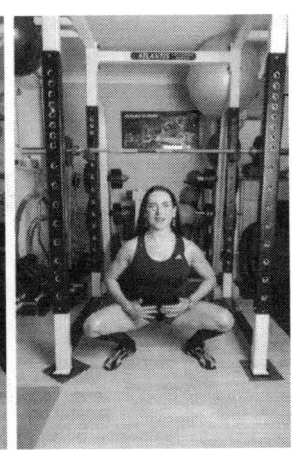

Starting Position   **¼ Squat**   **Full Squat**

Booty Bounce!

I learned this exercise from Pilates trainer, Lynne Robinson, UK , about 20 years ago. Simply lay on the floor on your back with legs in a "V" position (spread wide just outside hip width). Now begin pressing the heels into the floor and bounce your backside up and down very gently into the mat. Make sure you are on a soft comfortable mat and not a hard floor. Bounce gently. Don't slam! Inhale for 5 bounces and exhale for 5 bounces. Continue this for up to a minute, rest, take a break and repeat as often as you would like.

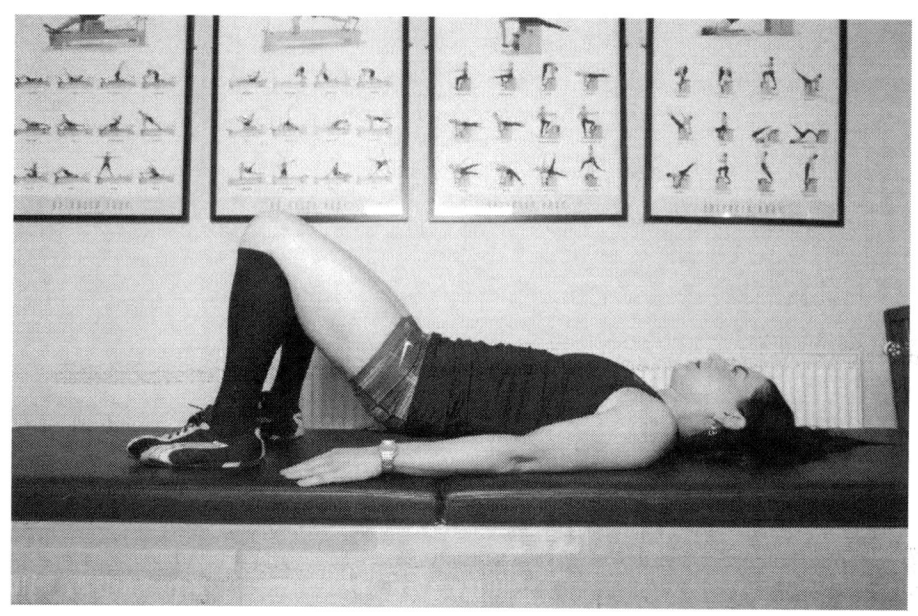

Booty bounce

Inner thigh pulse

Lie on your back and raise legs up as close to 90 degrees as possible (if you are very tight in the hamstrings bend your knees). Now as you inhale open the legs as wide as flexibility allows. Exhale as you close the legs in. Keep a continuous activation of the zip up of your pelvic floor. Inhale to open and exhale to close. You can try a long range and a short range of this exercise.

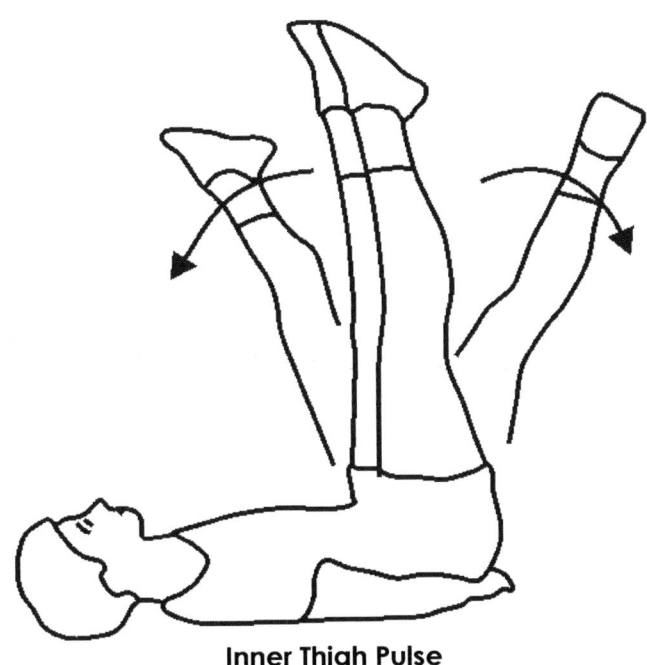
Inner Thigh Pulse

Pelvic Floor Squeezes

All of the pelvic floor exercises can be used as bioenergy ones. See the strengthening exercises chapter.

Glute Squeeze

The buttock squeeze from the previous chapter also works very well as a bioenergy exercise. Try it seated standing and laying down on your stomach, or laying down on your back.

Hip lift on the floor

Lay on your back with the legs in the "V" position just outside of the hips. Squeeze butt as you press heels into the floor and then lift up the hips till knees, hips and shoulders are in a straight line. Pulse up and down never fully landing the butt. Exhale up and inhale down. Keep constant tension on the butt.

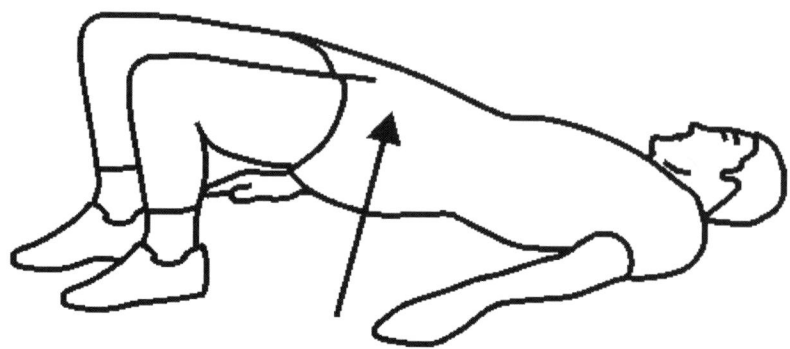

Hip lift on the floor

Buttock walk

This exercise is only for those with excellent hamstring length. Remember there are lots of other alternatives. Sit tall on the floor with long legs out in front. Now loco mote forwards on the butt, "walking" from one butt cheek to the other. Go for a certain length maybe 20 to 30 shuffles then reverse and go backwards. Keep the trunk upright.

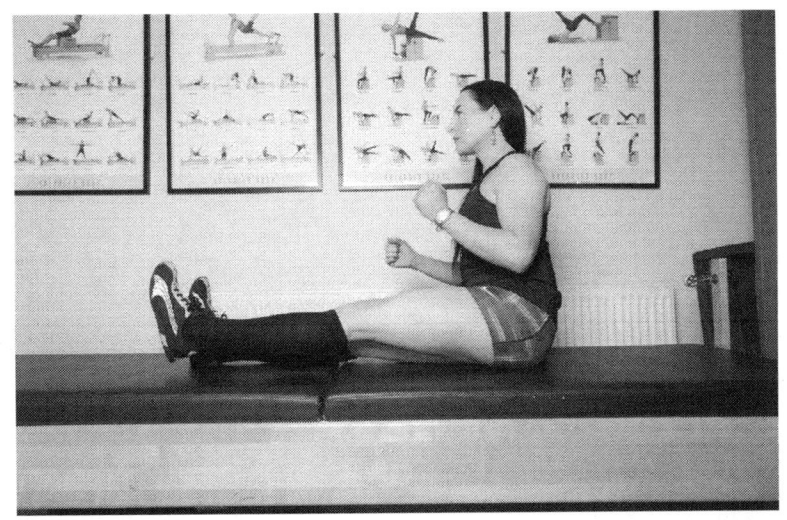

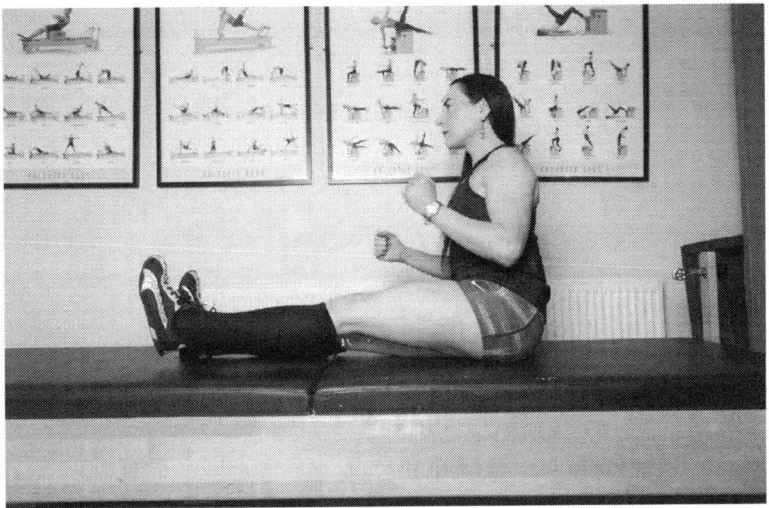

Buttock walk

Kneeling Squat

Kneel on a soft mat with knees slightly in a "V" position. Sit back on the heels. Now squeeze buttocks and come up to a position where the hips and knees are in alignment. Lower back to the start. Exhale up and inhale to lower.

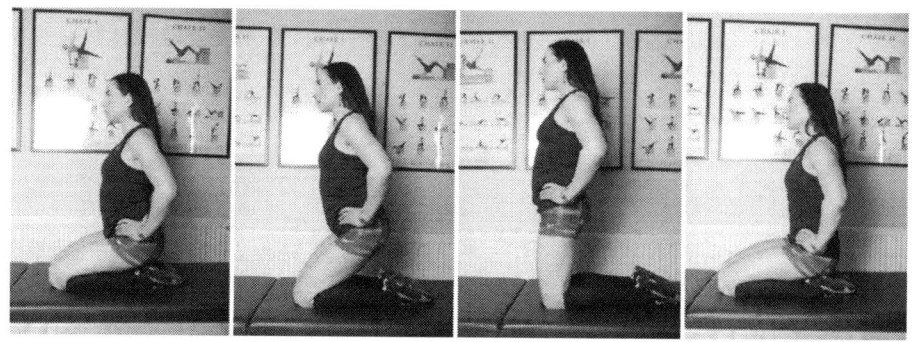

Kneeling squat

Shake and Vibrate

This is a technique to break down the holding patterns in the body. In western medicine we talk about scar tissue build up and fascial adhesions. In biomechanics we talk about flexibility restrictions.

Energetically it amounts to all of the decisions, judgements, conclusions and thoughts we have arrived at in our cognitive mind that lock up our reality and manifest as restrictions in the physical body. These restrictions also represent the toxic emotions (the lower harmonics of feeling) that we bought as real and true. In physiology this manifests as a trigger point, an area of restriction in a muscle that contains a mass of toxins.

In this exercise we are breaking down these old patterns by physically shaking the body out of the usual grooves it settles into. If we can change our point of view, get out of judgement and purify ourselves from these toxic emotions, the body can no longer hold onto the tension and lock down it is experiencing. Shaking the body is one of the most ancient forms of healing used by tribal peoples all over the planet most notably the Kalahari Bushmen. It's also used in Shamanic traditions.

To begin the exercise, start in a standing position with the feet just outside of the hips and arms resting by sides. Now start shaking the body swinging arms, letting the shoulders bob up and down. Let the knees remain soft. Move the body left and right. Shake the chest, shimmy the hips, experiment! If you are self-conscious don't do it in a public gym!

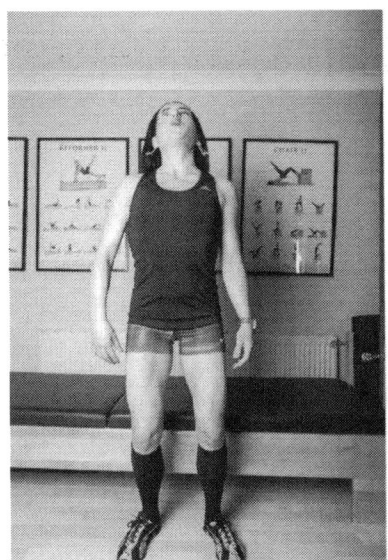 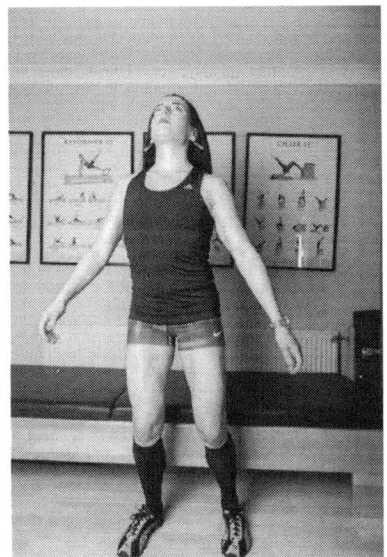

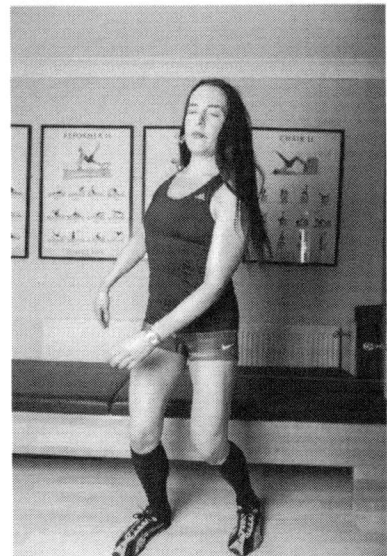

Root Chakra Hakka

This exercise is very loosely based on the Māori warrior dance made famous by the New Zealand All Blacks. Once again stand feet hip with apart, knees soft, arms relaxed by your side. Now do a mini jump and land slam style on your feet making a loud thud. Simultaneously make a loud cry like a warrior cry "Ha!" Let the sound come deep from your belly. Take a nice deep breath between jumps so the sound can be nice and powerful. Let your shoulders completely relax and leave your arms floppy.

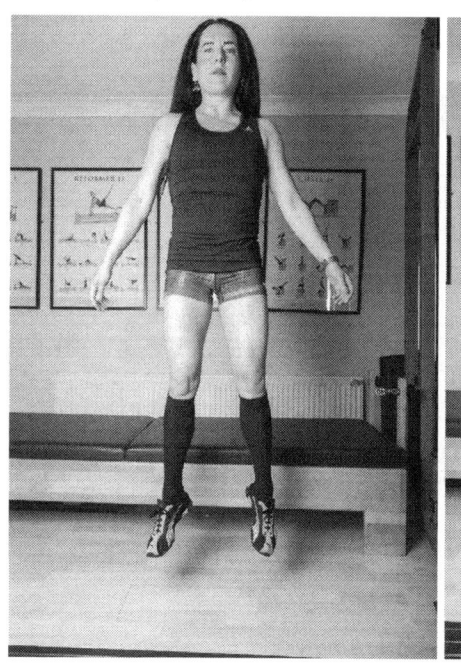 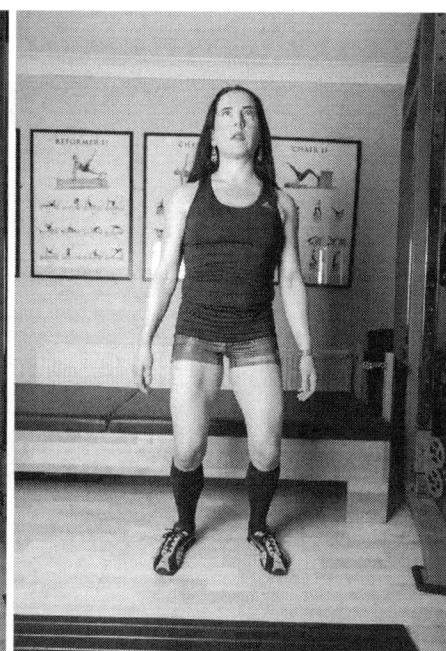

How to apply the exercises

Work your way through all of the exercises and see which ones give your body a sense of release or groundedness or extra vitality. All of these are indications that your base chakra is being stimulated. Remember you can't do it wrong as the energy has its own intelligence. Just use your power of intention together with your attention on the exercise in question and it will work a treat. You may find yourself drawn to one or two exercises in particular. Focus on these. I find myself being drawn to certain exercises more than others depending on what's going on in my body and in my life. Your body will love doing the exercises that work for it. Just make sure your mind does not get in the way. The acid test is to do the exercise for a few minutes and feel how the body reacts to it.

Chapter 9

Family systems and tribal/Ancestral contracts

The root chakra is also known as the base chakra. We hear people talking about going back to their roots or finding their roots. This usually has to do with a person returning to their home land (family or ancestral) or people exploring the family history or putting together a family tree. This phenomenon has recently been popularised by the BBC documentary "Who do you think you are?" where celebrities trace their family trees and find out some surprises.

Our family and ancestral/tribal associations have massive implications for not just our root chakra health but our entire lives. It includes things like our genetics, our cultural preferences, our religious and spiritual outlook on life, our beliefs about wealth/poverty and abundance/lack. We have expressions like "the apple does not fall far from the tree", "trust fund baby", "genetic freak", "like father, like son" that are a constant reminder of the pervasive influence our family and ancestors have on our lives.

The most important starting point in terms of one's wellbeing right now is to heal any trauma or drama surrounding your relationship with each parent.

There are many ways to do this from psychotherapy to spiritual coaching to group therapy like family systems therapy. If you do not heal your relationship with your parents individually, your relationship with your Mother and your relationship with your Father all of your relationships will play out the trauma and drama of this pain as your Being tries to resolve it. Many people would benefit from working with a professional in this area.

The foundation of our whole emotional lives comes from the experiences we hard during childhood. In the 1990s over 17,000 patients of a health care company were enrolled in a study to see the connections between their childhood experience and their current state of heath. It was called the ACE study (Adverse Childhood Experience). Those in the study who had experienced adverse conditions during childhood had between 4 and 50 times the risk of developing a serious health condition or disease. Questionnaires that were used in this study are available at:

http://www.cdc.gov/ace/questionnaires.htm

The adverse events included: having violent or abusive parents, witnessing physical or verbal abuse in the home, parents being alcoholic, not having clean clothes to wear, moving home frequently, sexual abuse and never having felt loved or wanted.

These events and the trauma that arose from them must be healed in order for the person to be well. There is an expression "the mind forgets but the body never forgets". We must gain access to the trauma and unresolved emotions that constitute the back log catalogue of our lives. This has been referred to as our cellular memory or "issues in our tissues". There are many techniques available today to assist people in unlocking this cellular memory.

Since everything is energy I have found that working through the chakras using energy exercises, food, nutrients and awareness exercises like observing the body and communicating with the body directly will unlock this stuck energy.

The Males energies; your relationship with your father

The Males energies represent the Yang side of the polarity. This has to do with:

Outward force and strength,

Outward appearances

Confidence

Doing

Work ethic

Taking action

Taking the steps to put things into place

Organisation

Planning

Goal setting

Giving direction/leadership

Taking care of the practical things

How this manifests in a man in a conventional male role within society and within the home would be as follows:

The man is the provider. He brings home the bacon so to speak. Going back to our caveman ancestors the males were the ones out hunting simply due to their superior physical size and strength. The man provided security by providing shelter and protection from harm.

How this would manifest in an individual regardless of their gender would be the ability to embody the traits listed above. So if you have a difficulty with confidence, planning and taking action or standing up for yourself maybe you need to look at your relationship with your Father.

Polarity; aligning and agreeing /resisting and reacting

Anything you align and agree with or resist and react to can become a problem. So if you align and agree with your fathers amazing work ethic you could become a workaholic just to prove how much you love your dad.

One of my dear clients in order to prove her love for her father went on to study a long and arduous degree and began working in a career she absolutely hated. She developed serious pain symptoms all down the right leg (the male or yang side of the body). This job was the one deemed by her father to provide the most security but because it was not working for her on a soul level (she was by no means passionate about it) it was literally destroying her health and thus her happiness.

On the other hand if we resist and react to our father's way of being in the world or his choices then we will push these elements out of our world unless we become aware of the pattern. So if your father was wealthy and you resented it because he spent so much time working and you didn't see him very often as a child, you may be pushing money and abundance out of your life! Is that really working for you?

Exercise:

Write down all of the ways that you have aligned and agreed with your father AND all of the ways you have resisted and reacted to him. Now go and erase everything on each list vibrationally e.g." Everything that my list brings up I now erase" or "everything on my list I now cancel, clear and delete" You can say this out loud or to yourself. Saying it out loud is more powerful. Whichever phrase sits best with you will work fine. You can't erase, cancel or delete the truth; you can only erase lies and limitation.

You can also erase or delete your relationship with your father every day. This is not as crazy as it sounds. It's just an energetic way of wiping the slate clean on all of the stuff that isn't working for you (or him!) in your relationship.

The Female energies: your relationship with your Mother

The female energies represent the Yin side of the equation. These qualities are embodied by the following:

Rest and relaxation

Dreaming

Creativity

Nurturing

Care, Love, Kindness

Sensuality

Artistry

Emotional support

Feeling

Perceiving

Being

If your mother was embodying the classical female model she would have stayed at home, tended the house, baked and prepared meals, read bed time stories, rubbed your knee when you had a fall, gave you hugs and lots of tactile interaction. She would have been the nurturer and carer and provider of emotional support. In the modern world many women are out working outside of the home through necessity or choice.

Hence the feminine role model within the household may not have been obvious.

Perhaps the mother was too busy to spend time nurturing and caring for the child's emotional development. This comes from spending time with children, listening to them, asking and answering questions, playing with them, being tactile with hugs and physical contact. This is incredibly important to the emotional development of the child. Children who are brought up in an environment devoid of physical contact show high levels of stress hormones like cortisol in their blood stream even up to 4 years after they have been placed in a home. Also their hormones associated with bonding like oxytocin and vasopressin were compromised[1].

A child perceives the world not intellectually but through feeling and if it is not feeling loved and wanted it is devastating to its development. This is the foundation stone of a person's self-esteem.

Children are the psychic sponge bobs of the Universe. They soak up all of the energetic information around them. If they perceive vibrations of anger, rage, hatred, blame, shame, anxiety and depression or any other toxic emotion they can lock it into their bodies and misidentify the energy as theirs or they can act it out and appear to be "difficult children". In reality they may be acting out the suppressed anger, fear and anxiety of the people around them.

Healing your relationship with your Mother

Write down all of the ways that you have aligned and agreed with your Mother and all of the ways you have resisted and reacted to her i.e. the things you like about her and the things you don't like. It's a known fact that people who hate their Mothers turn out exactly like them!

If we align and agree with something or resist and react to something we will manifest that very behaviour or way of being within ourselves. Now your life is no longer yours. You are living someone else's life. Is that really working for you? Are you going to allow your Mother to become the limitation on the type of person you can become or the level of achievement and happiness you will allow yourself to have?

Once you have made out your list now erase or cancel/clear/delete both the alignment and agreement parts and the resistance and reaction parts. By aligning and agreeing or resisting and reacting to something or someone you become polarised. That is you become split in two. All healing is about healing this illusory split. What causes this split? The answer is judgement. When you judge something you take sides. You align and agree or you resist and react. Either way you lose because you disintegrate yourself. If you align and agree or resist and react to your Mother you separate yourself from yourself. All healing is a healing of the illusion of separation.

This principle is one of the foundation stones of all Spiritual traditions. It is also supported by Quantum Physics. Everything is connected by the energetic matrix of the universe. Everything is energy. Energy is not good or bad it just has different frequency. The cosmos does not judge energy. There is space for all energies.

Just like you did with your Father erase or delete your relationship with your Mother every day. This will help also to erase the memory of all hurt or slights and the relationship has the space to grow and evolve into something that is a greater contribution to your life.

Genetics and Epigenetics

The word Genetics comes from Genesis meaning origin. Our genetics are a series of codes that convey our traits. This encoding is handed down through the DNA/RNA structures. Many people think that genetics are the be all and end all of our physical health and what is possible for us with respect to physical endeavour and intellectual prowess. Many people fear their genes and see them as a potential threat if they inherit "bad genes". But this is simply not the case.

Genetics represent a potential outcome and not an absolute one. There are two phenomena that one must consider when dealing with genetics and that is the difference between a genotype and phenotype. The genotype is the exact genes you inherited from your parents. These genes are carried on 23 pairs of chromosomes. 23 chromosomes come from the father and 23 come from the mother giving you about 25,000 genes!

Whether a gene gets to program a result depends on many factors including dominant and recessive genes and the chemical/behavioural environment of the genes (epigenetics). What actually shows up is known as the phenotype. E.g. you could receive genes for blue eyes from your mother and brown eyes from your father and what shows up are brown eyes. Your phenotype is brown eyes.

The expression "Genetics loads the gun and the Environment pulls the trigger" is very fitting. Supplying the body with excellent nutrition and adopting healthy lifestyle including techniques shared in this book can literally alter the destiny of your genetic programming. For example you could have genes that predispose you to obesity but by adopting a healthy lifestyle, training with weights in a progressive manner and eating in a way to support fat loss and maintain lean body mass you will never be obese.

"It's estimated that as little as 10% and no more than 25% of your personal health is determined by your genetics"

Dr Bob Rackowski

In a landmark study titled "Epigenetic programming by maternal behaviour", which was published in the Journal Nature Neuroscience in June 2004 , researchers clearly demonstrated the potential of the environment to create changes in genes expression of an unfavourable kind[2]. In the study two different environments were tested with regard to the parenting of baby rats. In one group there was lots of licking, preening and snuggling under the mother's belly. In the other group there was significantly less of this tactile interaction. The poor unfortunate rats that did not have that loving touch began to get significant methylation of their DNA in the brain regions responsible for stress response, namely the hippocampus. They now had a heightened stress response. Other studies have shown increase of this phenomenon in suicide cases. Some more recent research links chronic pain to epigenetic changes in the brain:

"Injury results in long-term changes to the DNA markings in the brain; our work shows it might be possible to reverse the effects of chronic pain by interventions using either behavioural or pharmacological means that interfere with DNA methylation. Our findings have the potential to completely alter the way we treat chronic pain."

Prof. Szyf , McGill University

The bottom line remains your DNA is not your destiny. Nutrients, environmental factors and even behavioural factors can reshape the expression of those genes for better or for worse.

Genetic Testing

Although genetics do not determine the entire fate of your health, they most certainly have an influence. In recent years genetic testing has become more widely available to the general public. What are the benefits?

Genetic risk factors for disease

One of the most obvious benefits is that you can find out if you have an increased risk for certain types of cancer. Hereditary breast and ovarian cancer is mediated by the BRAC1 and BRAC2 genes respectively. Mutations of these genes can lead to a substantial increased risk of developing the above cancers. Knowing about this can help people make decisions that may be lifesaving.

Drug response

Your genetics can reveal how drugs react in your body. This may help a doctor to make a more appropriate decision when deciding a course of drug treatment for a given condition.

Traits

One of the traits that your genes can reveal is how quickly you metabolise caffeine from your body. Individuals who are slow metabolisers can significantly increase their risk of heart attack by drinking as little as two cups a day. Individuals who have a gene variant that allows for rapid caffeine clearance may actually reduce their heart attack risk by drinking coffee[3]. Considering how popular this beverage is and how prevalent heart disease is, this could be some very useful information indeed!

Even how your body responds to exercise and the type of diet that can work best for you can be indicated by your genes. This information could really assist the individual fine tuning their exercise and nutritional plan.

The Downsides of Genetic Testing

While many interesting pieces of information can be garnered from genetic testing, there are downsides. There may be unfavourable emotional consequences to finding out ones genetic weaknesses. It could create upset among other family members. Family secrets may be exposed. It has the potential to possibly affect insurance policies. All of these things need to be considered before proceeding.

For more information on genetic testing see:

www.23andme.com

Ancestral Patterns and Morphic Resonance

The next few items that I am going to discuss are not as concrete as DNA, genes and chromosomes, the physical inheritance from our ancestors. New theories suggest that we also inherit thought patterns, feelings, emotions and beliefs from our ancestors. These patterns of organisation are called Morphic fields (A theory by Rupert Sheldrake).

So if your Ancestors had beliefs about poverty and struggle for example you may be unwittingly pulled into a Morphic field (an energy field comprised of thoughts, feelings, beliefs, decisions, judgements and conclusions on a given topic) that causes you to generate and create a constant experience of poverty in your life. Your root chakra is your chakra of manifestation. So if you are "doing the leg work" and taking action to create abundance and wealth in your life and nothing you do seems to work maybe you are being influenced by these Morphic fields. You can visualise yourself unplugging from the Morphic fields that no longer serve you.

Visualisation to unplug from Morphic Fields

Get in a nice comfortable position with your spine aligned and upright. Close your eyes and take a few deep breaths allowing your belly to expand and relax. Ask your Infinite Being (that part of you that is constantly connected to Source, sometimes called Higher Self or Christ Self) to show you all of the Morphic fields you are plugging into that are blocking the flow of abundance and prosperity in your life. You may now get a visual image if you are a visual person or maybe a feeling or sensation. Ask your Infinite Being to unplug you from these Morphic fields and move you into new Morphic Fields of abundance and prosperity.

Again if you are visual you may see an image of this happening or you or you may feel sensations. Trust that it is happening. Ask and you shall receive is a basic principle of the Universe. This trust will stabilise your base chakra even more as it eliminates fear. The more you practice this (and it can take just a few minutes) the more you move to abundance and prosperity.

Are Morphic Fields a new phenomenon?

The term Morphic field may be relatively new but the principle behind it is not. At the most basic level Man is an animal and many of his/her behaviours are conditioned by what is known as the pack instinct. The pack (animal) or Tribal (human) instinct was meant to be one that enhanced the survival of the individual and the species as a whole.

Take a look at a flock of flamingos and their behaviour. If a predator comes and startles one of them the bird breaks into flight. Almost instantaneously all of the flock will lift off at almost the same time. This response is way too fast to be a standard reflex. One possible theory to explain this is the Morphic Field theory. Every flamingo would be connected into the Morphic Field of the flock. When one got a fright the other members of the flock would get a fright at the exact same time.

Even quantum physics seems to be veering away from particulate description of the universe (atoms, molecules, protons etc.) to one where fields of energy are described:

"Many physicists think that particles are not things at all but excitations in a quantum field, the modern successor of classical fields such as the magnetic field" [4].

So maybe we are not as separate as we appear. We have expressions such as *zeitgeist which* literally means spirit of the age.

"No man can surpass his own time, for the spirit of his time is also his own spirit."

German philosopher Georg Hegel

We also have the term "collective consciousness" originally coined by the French sociologist Emile Durkheim in 1893. This term refers to a sort of group awareness or shared perception.

Whether the theories are very new and somewhat controversial (morphic field theory) , well established in modern science (quantum Field theory), or originated with musings on human behaviour many fields of study continue to point to our inherent interconnectedness, an interconnectedness that runs deeper than belonging to the same species or tribe.

Healing your family issues give you a great footing for the rest of your life. You have that rock solid foundation on which to build upon. We have the expression; "He/She didn't have a leg to stand on" denoting a situation where a person has no chance. Our relationship with our Father is the foundation stone or leg for our thinking world or the world of mind. Our relationship with our Mother is the foundation stone for our feeling world or body. We require a solid footing in both worlds or else the weak footing will become the limiting factor.

If you refuse to identify which parent you have issues with (you usually have issues with both but one may be more challenging than the other) you will find yourself attracting in relationships and friendships that play out the drama and trauma of these relationships.

Those interactions/relationships will continuously knock you off your seat of power. You will battle the person in question in an attempt to resolve the original wound of the parent in question. If you do not see the cycle and pattern you just keep attracting in new people with the same story and message. And usually that message gets louder and louder and possibly more dramatic and traumatic.

Heal your relationship with both parents and your root chakra will strengthen.

Ancestral Karma

"Nothing influences children more than the silent facts in the background"[5]

Carl Jung

Beyond the physical inheritance of genes and the inheritance of beliefs and talents many schools of thought from Western Psychology to Eastern Yogic traditions have a concept of inheriting unfinished business from their ancestors.

The hidden, unspoken and unacknowledged secrets, traumas and dramas of our ancestors can play out in our psyches so fully that we believe they are our own. These patterns are thought to be the root cause of patterns like Alcoholism, Addictions, Depression, Mental Illness, Incest and other issues of Abuse.

"For I the Lord your God am a jealous God, visiting iniquity of the fathers on the children to the 3rd and 4th generations of those who hate me."[6]

The Bible

"The sins of the father are to be laid upon the children"[7]

William Shakespeare

"We are all metabolizing our ancestral legacy of subtle or overt abuse which has been passed down and propagated throughout the generations"[8]

Paul Levey

How can these so called sins be passed down from one generation to the next? The answer may lie in what Carl Jung termed "Participation mystique". This is a phenomenon whereby we become enmeshed and entangled in the hidden grief and unresolved trauma of another person's consciousness e.g. a child can perceive all of the unconscious and unresolved mental and emotional content of a parent and they assume that it's theirs. Let's say you grow up in a household where your mother is depressed, as a child you perceive all of your mothers projected and unresolved mental and emotional baggage and reach the conclusion that you are also depressed. This depression is not yours but you have made it yours by a misinterpretation of your awareness of your surroundings. You have been unable to differentiate your feelings from your Mothers feelings. You have purchased her story and unresolved trauma as yours.

Getting Free of Ancestral Karma

1: Family Constellations Therapy.

This is one method of approaching the clearing of your ancestral karma. It is based on the work of Bert Hellinger. People who have trained in his system set up family constellations and work in group sessions or private sessions to help you unfold any family issue from your current family to your ancestors. Other family members need not be present. To find a facilitator for this work go to: http://www2.hellinger.com

2: Ritual

In many cultural traditions throughout the world Ancestors are honoured by specific rituals. The festival of Halloween was originally one where our ancestors were remembered and honoured. In certain yogic traditions alters are made to honour the ancestors and offerings of food are left there.

Visiting a deceased loved ones grave would be an example of a healing and honouring ritual that most Westerners would be familiar with.

In Shamanic traditions fire ceremonies are held in honour of the ancestors.

Chapter 10

Mindfulness about your Behaviour

Certain behaviours both functional and dysfunctional come under the governance of the root chakra. In reading through these you will understand why over 90% of the world's population has a dysfunctional root chakra. Step one of changing a problem is to become aware of it. In the highest level of truth nothing is a problem as everything is here to assist our growth and a return to the recognition of the Divine Perfection that we all are.

Responsibility

Responsibility is a phenomenon of the root chakra. Ever heard the expression "Stand on your own two feet"? Well that simply means take responsibility for yourself. We are all master creators of our own reality. Through our thoughts, feelings, beliefs and actions we create every nuance of our life experience.

We are the writer, director, starring character and editor in the movie of our own lives. We cast all of the other characters in our movie. We have written the script! And if we don't like the script as directors we can change it at any moment. Nobody can do anything to you! Nobody can make you feel, think or do anything. You are responsible for all of it.

Responsibility for many feels like a heavy, loaded term. In reality it is the path to freedom. Responsibility is the "ability to respond". No matter what happens deep down I know I have the power to respond to all situations. My whole Being has been designed to cope with every possible scenario that comes my way. I may need to remind myself of this very often so that I can stand in my power at all times. One of the mantras that I use when I am doing heavy squats is "I AM the Power and the Might!" We would do well to remind ourselves of this as often as is required.

When you do not realise that you are the creator and director of your whole life experience you become a victim of circumstance. Another way of phrasing this is that you abdicate responsibility. Life just happens to you. You have "bad luck". Other people "make you do stuff or feel stuff". Ever seen toddlers in a fight over something? One little kid hits another and the response is he/she made me do it! Adults still do this all the time! "You made me angry!", "I couldn't help myself" and " I had no choice". All of these phrases are the battle cry of one who has no intention of taking responsibility.

One of the areas that this plays out very obviously is in the creation of our own bodies. If we are not willing to take responsibility for the type and quality of the food we put into our mouths, the exercise we do or don't do our emotional wellness and self-care our bodies will show up as the living testament to this lack of responsibility.

People who are not willing to take responsibility think they can pay somebody else to take responsibility for them. I have witnessed this phenomenon very often in my role as a personal trainer. Somebody rocks up and pays you for a couple of training sessions a week in order to "whip them into shape". All the while the person in question does not follow their nutritional plan, binges at the weekend, over consumes alcohol, refuses to do the inner work required , and ignores any and all advice given. This person has no intention to change.

Transformation of the body and Being can be a very painful, arduous and long process. There is nothing comfortable about it. If you are not willing to go into the discomfort of passing on the biscuits at break time or feeling all of your suppressed anger come to the surface on a liver cleanse you are not willing to be responsible. If you are not willing to be responsible you will play the role of victim and blame others or circumstances for your lack of success or you will keep putting off the things, you know you could be doing, that would create change i.e. you procrastinate.

Nobody is responsible for your body, your life or your success as a human being. You are doing it all. You are creating it all. The road to freedom starts with personal responsibility. You need to get back on this road daily, sometimes hourly and sometimes moment to moment. Remember you can't pay anybody to live your life for you. Now stand on your own two feet and be the power and the might that you came here to be!

Self-Respect

There are a lot of definitions out there as regards to what Self –Respect is. My personal definition is linked to the root chakra which is all about taking action. It's also linked to trust. So for me Self-Respect is trusting that I both know and am able to take the appropriate action to honour myself in all possible situations.

E.g. I respect my body so I feed it foods that honour its requirements and I participate in exercise that I enjoy and that honours how my body functions and what my body requires to be strong and healthy.

People with no self-respect use their bodies as a garbage disposal unit eating foods that do not honour the body's innate desire to feel healthy and well. People who have no self-respect abuse their bodies with either no exercise or excessive exercise that totally beats the body up. Unfortunately this is endemic in the modern world, with excessive exercise and brutal regimens where participants frequently get injured or burn themselves out totally.

When I have self-respect I surround myself with people who treat me well and honour me as a person. I trust myself to know when a relationship or behaviour is damaging to me and I remove myself from the situation. E.g. in a relationship setting if a "friend" is always putting you down you respect yourself by standing up for yourself (another root chakra metaphor). If the behaviour continues you trust yourself to end that friendship or relationship.

People with no self-respect become the doormats of the universe. Pablo Picasso famously said:

"There are only two types of women – goddesses and doormats."

The same scenario can of course be applied to men.

People can develop issues around self-respect if they grew up in an environment where one parent constantly disrespected the other or they were directly disrespected by one or both parents or if they were bullied by siblings or peers.

How we allow ourselves to be treated largely depends on what our life experience was in the formative years of our lives. So if we are a young child experiencing violence in the home the fear response will come up telling us to get the hell out of there. When we have self- respect we honour and trust this feeling. However where can you go if you are a child?

Many people who have come from abusive backgrounds with alcoholic or violent parents need to do a lot of work to repair their self-respect- their ability to trust themselves enough to take appropriate action to honour themselves.

How do you know if a person has self-respect? Simply observe how they allow themselves to be treated.

Co-Dependency

When you stand on your own two feet you stand in your own power and everything you require comes to you. The opposite of this is looking outside of your-self for this sense of power. One can look to other people, substances (alcohol, drugs etc.) or situations (e.g. work) to bring this feeling. This feeling we crave can be a sense of belonging, fitting in (all tribal root chakra associations) and feeling needed. If we are not sustained by our own lifeline (the root chakra runs from the pelvic floor like an energetic line to the centre of the earth) we look to others (people, situations, substances) to try to get the energy we require there.

People from abusive backgrounds are classic candidates who become co-dependent. In fact most people are co-dependent in some way and this is not healthy. Anytime you look outside of yourself in any way to have your needs met it is some form of co-dependence.

All addictions are a form of co-dependence. A relationship whereby one person looks after another person's needs at the expense of their own is a co-dependence.

If you are not able or willing to take responsibility for yourself you may feel inordinately responsible for other people. That is also co-dependence.

Other signs of co-dependence include:

Low self esteem

Lack of self confidence

Inappropriate boundaries; too many or none at all

Being the doormat of the universe

Not being able to say no

Always wanting your own way

Being a control freak

Manipulating others or being the victim of manipulation

All forms of addiction (drugs, alcohol, shopping, sex, gambling.)

Staying in a relationship way past its sell by date

Trying to change people

Looking to others to gauge your value or worth in the world

Neediness -The co-dependent is both the needy person and the person trying to take care of everybody else's needs while abandoning their own.

Rescuing others

Fixing others

Wanting to change others

The co-dependent has deep emotional wounds that they avoid looking at by focusing on others dysfunctionalism.

At the root of the issue the co-dependent has safety and security issues stemming from a fear of abandonment.

Most co-dependents will be recommended professional counselling to identify and modify their behaviour.

Simply by working through the exercises in this book one can strengthen the root chakra so much that many co-dependent behaviours may fall away.

One of my clients took up strength training with me so that she would have the strength to walk away from a bad marriage. On a subconscious level she knew that if she was physically strong it would support the mental and emotional strength required to face change.

Persons with a weak root chakra always fear change.

Energetic Exercise to Cut the Cords of Co-Dependency

Persons with severe co-dependent issues like alcoholism, drug addiction and being in an abusive relationship are of course recommended professional support through a group like alcoholics anonymous, co-dependants anonymous or a professional therapist.

The following is an energetic technique to disconnect inappropriate attachments to persons, substances and situations that do not serve our highest good and wellbeing.

Sit with your spine upright on your sits bones. Breathe deeply in through the nose and out through the mouth. Visualise a beam of light dropping from your pelvic floor down to the centre of the earth. Visualise another beam going out from the top of your head up to the heavens. Visualise both beams of light connecting at your heart centre. Now there is one beam of white light connecting you from the heavens to the earth through your heart centre.

Now say the following to yourself:

"I now ask my infinite Being (Higher Consciousness, Christ Self) to show me all of the Cords, Hooks, Ties and attachments binding me to other Persons, Substances, or Situations that no longer serve my path of greatest Harmony and Health. "

You may get awareness through feeling, sensation or visual image.

Now continue by saying:

"Disconnect all"

You may add a visualisation of guillotine blades coming down on all sides' disconnection all of the cords, hooks, ties and attachments. Continue visualising the white light flowing through you top to bottom filling up your whole body. Imagine the white light dislodging any of the roots of these cords, hooks, ties and attachments and incinerating them on the spot.

You can now visualise your Aura totally filled up with pure white radiant light from the highest of the high. Your Aura is Egg shaped and extends a few feet outside your body. Now visualise a golden tube of light surrounding this egg shaped Aura which represents appropriate interpersonal boundaries.

You may finish the visualisation/meditation with the statement

"And so IT IS".

For further reading on the topic of co-dependency see the excellent book:

Co-dependency For Dummies by Darlene Lancer, JD, MFT

Eating –Disorders

The body requires food to survive and all survival issues are a base chakra phenomenon. The aetiology of eating disorders has nothing to do with food as such. Food is just a symptom. The person with the eating disorder had some disturbance in their energetic field that caused the root chakra to become dysfunctional. Usually the individual is trying to avoid intensely painful emotions like fear, feeling unsafe, guilt and shame. Many individuals who manifest an eating disorder like anorexia nervosa for example have been abused in some way:

"In my eating disorder practice, 40 to 60 percent of the men and women who come to therapy for an eating problem have been sexually or physically abused"

Mary Anne Cohen, CSW, Director – The New York Centre for Eating Disorders

Since the root chakra is the safety and security chakra and also the chakra of the primal urge for sex and the chakra of trust all forms of abuse have a severe damaging effect on this chakra. The abuse of trust can be so severe that one cannot trust ones instinct to eat for survival.

Eating disorders are notoriously difficult to treat and have the highest death rate of all mental disorders. Not surprising when one considers that the health of the root chakra supplies our "will to live "

When a person is abused it's as if their power is taken away. Their boundaries have been seriously breached. The behaviour around food then becomes a quest to be "in control" at all times. This feeling of control does two things: It numbs out the deep traumatic feelings and it gives the person in question a sense of safety.

The opposite to control is surrender. This is not to be confused with an apathetic abandonment of life but surrender to the trust that the universe and the process of life has your back.

By not eating one avoids being present in the body and when one is not fully present the difficult feelings cannot be felt. The root chakra is the chakra of the present moment. It really represents the power of NOW. In order to fully be present in the now all past trauma needs to be resolved.

Special treatment programs are available for persons with eating disorders however many do not get to this stage as they are either in denial or they resist treatment.

By practicing the energetic exercises in this book one may generate a foundational energy that would allow the person to take the next step in their recovery.

Research from the Stanford University School of Medicine has shown that Family based therapy, in which the parents of adolescents with the disease were enlisted in the therapy process, was twice as effective as individual based psychotherapy. James Lock MD PhD was one of the main leaders of this research. The root chakra is connected to family and tribal issues. Anything that supports the root chakra could in theory help a given individual.

Anorexia nervosa may also have a physiological component. Research from as early as the 1970s shows that Zinc deficiency is a key player in the onset of the disease. Zinc is connected with the production of testosterone, our appetite regulation and sense of smell and taste to name but a few.

This therapy may work for certain individuals and needs to be done under the supervision of a health care practitioner. A multi-pronged approach of counselling and nutritional therapy and bio-energetic exercise is best.

Addictions

Another symptom of dysfunction at the root chakra is addictions. Addictions are a symptom of trying to alleviate pain and discomfort when our most basic needs are not being met. Our brain function at base chakra level is all about the 3 s's: Safety, Sustenance and Sex. We need to feel safe, we need to have a full belly and we need to satisfy our carnal desires for sex. All of these 3 come under the control of what is known as our reptilian brain (first identified by American physician and neuroscientist Paul D MacLean).

Dopamine; the neurotransmitter of Motivation and Drive!

The root chakra component of addictions centres around the neurotransmitter Dopamine (the second part of the addictive equation relates to the neurotransmitter serotonin which is related to chakra II). Dopamine is the neurotransmitter of motivation and drive. It is the call to action! When we are stressed by safety, sustenance and sex issues dopamine is released. In an emergency situation dopamine can even be converted into adrenaline.

Chronic stress or unresolved feelings of being unsafe can deplete dopamine levels. Symptoms of low dopamine include: Lack of drive and motivation, fatigue, attention deficit disorder, low libido, addictive behaviour of all kinds, cravings and just feeling blah! At the most extreme level it manifests as Parkinson's disease which is a neuro-degenerative disease typified by a tremor of the hands.

In order to raise ones dopamine levels naturally a protein rich diet is recommended, meat, fish and eggs being the best sources. Beets, another root chakra food can boost dopamine via their betaine content. Coffee is also a stimulator of dopamine. I was interviewing a client one morning and she was telling me that she had a rare genetic disorder called Segawa Syndrome and that the only thing that prevented episodes was coffee. She said "Oh I know I shouldn't drink it!" On telling me she was on Parkinson's Meds I knew her body craved the coffee to produce dopamine (the exact same thing that the medication for Parkinson's does). If she was listening to what her brain was telling her as opposed to what her body knew would be medicinal, then she would have to take more medication instead of a natural food.

Tyrosine is one of the key amino acids that is a precursor to dopamine production. Foods highest in tyrosine include spirulina, eggs, cottage cheese, salmon and turkey.

One of the chemicals that breaks down dopamine is a substance called Mono Amine Oxidase or MAO for short. Some doctors prescribe MAO inhibitors for depressed patients to allow their dopamine levels to rebuild. Natural MAO inhibitors can be found in nature in the form of some spices, most notably nutmeg, passion flower and kava.

Supplements that support dopamine production include:

Tyrosine

DL-Phenylalanine

Mucuna Purines

One must approach supplementation with care. Too much dopamine is as bad as too little and is linked to lack of impulse control and even violence. Certain supplements are contraindicated for pregnant women or those already on MAO inhibiting medication. Consult your health care practitioner or doctor to assess suitability.

Safety/Security

One of the reptilian brains primary drives is that of survival. At the root of our being anything that threatens our survival or safety is one of our greatest terrors. Security and safety comes from two main wings; the Masculine or Yang side and the Feminine or Yin side. One way that we feel safe is when our physical needs are met in the form of food, shelter and protection. These are classically provided by the male energies.

The second form of security that must not be overlooked is the security that comes from being loved and nurtured in a tactile, vocally affirmative and motherly way. Of course this is provided classically by the female energies. Remember the study about the rats that were not licked and cuddled by their mothers? They developed derangements in their DNA due to this lack of feminine security.

This feminine security can be summed up in a nut shell; we desire to know and feel that we are loved. Research in orphanages has shown that lack of physical contact can increase mortality rates in young babies.

"Babies who are not held and nuzzled and hugged enough will literally stop growing and-if the situation lasts long enough, even if they are receiving proper nutrition- die. " [1]

At the root of most people's emotional issues is a severe lack of safety, coming from one or both sides of the security spectrum mentioned above.

If either parent is violent or prone to aggressive outbursts this can create a sense of severe security deficit in a child leading to post traumatic stress disorder. The child becomes hyper vigilant and produces so many stress hormones that their brain becomes rewired and remodelled to copper fasten the stress response. They are always on guard and may become reclusive or socially inept.

If the child does not receive the tactile hugs and physical nurturing they require methylation of their DNA may occur setting the stage for depression and low self-esteem.

The ultimate safety of course comes not from what we did or did not experience during childhood. It comes from the power of the present moment. In the present moment I can provide for myself and I can love and care for myself. In the present moment it is safe for me to experience the human condition.

New thought process:

If I trust and fully surrender to the present moment. All experiences can be transformed.

Crime/Violence

Crime and violence arise from the issues of safety and security. If someone is afraid they are unworthy or unlovable they can act it out in violent ways. If someone is afraid for their survival they can turn to crime.

> *"Violence is Fear in action"*
> *Matt Kahn*

Porn

Porn is the most primal drive for sex, it is lust without feeling. An addiction to porn or compulsivity about it is a sign of a dysfunctional root chakra. Many of these dysfunctions on a subconscious level are an attempt to drive energy to the root chakra. The most common symptom I have seen over the last 10 years is blocked or low energy in the root chakra. Many individuals become addicted to porn because they don't feel safe in their body's or in the world and an orgasm gives them temporary relief from the fear they are not even aware that they have. Research from Groningen University in the Netherlands has shown that the region of the brain that controls emotions like fear and anxiety (the amygdala) is suppressed during orgasm[2].

Over-Eating

Eating for some people provides a sense of security and safety. Every time you eat for example you mitigate the effects of stress hormones like cortisol. Eating certain foods in excess like sugars and grain based refined carbohydrate can create a feeling of emotional security. That warm fuzzy feeling of a serotonin rush. Unfortunately this feeling is transient. If we don't get these two wings of safety in an internal way we will perpetually chase the external salve. This for many is the real true cause of their obesity. Safety issues that are unresolved are being inappropriately treated with food. Food for many is the ultimate numbing device.

Control

Control is in fact the opposite of safety. When I am feeling safe there is nothing to control. In order to return to safety we surrender to what is. Again not in an apathetic self-defeated way but in a way which allows trust to return. All control freaks have safety and security issues, either from the Yin or Yang sides of security.

Examples of control freak behaviour:

Obsessive Compulsive Disorder

Orthorexia

Any form of eating that's overly disciplined or rigid

A belief that one's way of eating is THE WAY!!

Very scheduled daily activities

 Extreme structure

Never able to miss a work-out

No flexibility regarding way of living or being in the world

Always wanting your own way

No tolerance for other peoples point of view

Dogmatic beliefs

Trying to control others

Being a bossy boots!

If you notice that this is you -here are a few suggestions:

1. Try to shake up your routine a bit even if it just means driving a different route to work.

2. Try to blend your nutritional knowledge with biofeedback. Ask your body what it wants as opposed to dictating to it what your mind has decided it needs.

3. If you have been over zealous with your work outs don't be afraid to take some time off or switch to more Yin building activities for a while (e.g. bio-energetic exercises).

4. Let your friend or partner decide what movie to watch or which restaurant to visit.

5. Respect other people's perspective. Remember there is no right and wrong just differing points of view.

"There is no right and wrong, but thinking makes it so"
William Shakespeare

6. Try to introduce some more flow and spontaneity into your life.

Procrastination

Procrastination is the practice of putting things off till tomorrow or next week or "sometime when I have more time". The person in reality is too scared to take action. When we step up to take action in any area of our lives we move into a state of expansion. Our world gets bigger. During this process of expansion the controls and fears and limitations that kept us at that level of awareness are broken down. As they are broken down we feel the fear. As you feel the fear it is transformed.

Are you a person who is always putting things off? Ask yourself: "what is the worst thing that could happen if I decide to do this?" Fear of failure is one of the major issues for many. Curiously fear of success is the driver for others. If you are successful you may attract more attention and this becomes a bigger fear than the original fear. Fear holds you in a vibrational box of limitation. Procrastination is the security guard on the door of this vibrational box.

Poverty Consciousness and Money Obsession

Money and attitudes towards money are themes of the root chakra. One can see that money and survival are intertwined. One needs money to put a roof over your head and bread on the table. These are basic reptilian brain requirements. People have been killed for money. People will prostitute themselves for money. People will disrespect themselves for money. There is a misconception that money will cure the root chakra deficiency.

I once had a client many years ago who typified the dysfunctional root chakra concerns with regard to money. He was very weak with no leg development and a pancake butt. He was always restless and could not focus for any length of time. He was always fidgeting and one could see signs of hyper vigilance. He could not even close his eyes during a hands on healing session! He was obsessed with money and the acquisition of wealth. During some of our conversations it came to light that this guy's father had him out working on the farm from a very early age, maybe as young as 3 or 4. I had the intuition that this guy never really had a childhood and that he learned that making money=security =my father will love me. He would never make enough money to feel the security of the love he felt he did not get from his father.

Poverty consciousness is another example of dis-ease around money. Persons with a poverty consciousness usually grew up in an environment of poverty and lack. Their parents struggled to make ends meet. Growing up with poverty is a survival threat. Often times these people, even if they end up accumulating wealth, cannot enjoy their money. They fear losing it. They can't spend it. These people are the quintessential "tight asses" of the world. Your buttocks are such a metaphor for so many issues of the root chakra! Maybe that is why we are living in an era of "booty" obsession. In the zeitgeist we are trying to crack the root chakra code!

People with a poverty consciousness can never throw anything out or give stuff away. Their homes are filled with clutter. De-cluttering your home could be one of the best things you could do to boost your money flow. It's also curiously great to boost your own energy flow as the root chakra governs our overall vitality and how energised we feel.

You have often heard that money is just energy. Boost the flow of this energy by implementing the strategies in this book to heal and repair your root chakra and watch what happens to your money flow!

Persons who have a dysfunctional root chakra will have to overcompensate by becoming workaholics to get the level of financial success they desire. Unfortunately this can deplete the physical body. My money obsessed client used to say to me:

"You spend your health to gain your wealth then spend your wealth to regain your health!"

Why not heal your root chakra and let the abundance flow into your life with ease doing work you love that energises you instead of exhausting you?

Fear of Death

"It is impossible that anything so natural, so necessary and so universal as death should ever have been designed by Providence as an evil to mankind"

Jonathan Swift

The words of Jonathan swift may provide some comfort however fear of death remains one of the most pervasive fears of the human condition.

You see the reptilian brain can have no concept of an afterlife and the only aspect of you that is afraid of death is the reptilian brain. In order to go beyond the fear of death one must go beyond the reptilian brain. At the crown chakra level of existence we are one with the infinite nature of the universe. We are the alpha and the omega simultaneously. Therefore death is merely a transition from one state of being into another. For those who have some platform of spiritual outlook on life this is easier to accept.

In order to address the fear of death it may be useful to do some reading on the subject.

I have found a number of books to be very insightful on the subject:

After Life: the complete guide to life after death by Carol Neiman and Emily Goldman

The Tibetan book of the Living and the Dying by Sogyal Rinpoche

And

Proof of heaven: a neurosurgeon's journey into the afterlife. By Dr Eben Alexander

It should also be noted that thousands of people all over the world have had a "Near Death Experience". The stories of these individuals seem very hopeful indeed.

One person who has had this experience is the Irish Mystic and seer of angels Lorna Byrne:

"I know that I and others have all been given near death experiences so as we can share our experience and make people understand that death is not to be feared and that Heaven is real."

Another very inspiring lady who had a most profound near death experience is Anita Moorjani. She was diagnosed with a terminal cancer and given 36 hours to live. She wavered between two worlds during a coma like state and had the most profound experience. On awakening she made a miraculously recovery and within weeks all of her cancer was gone.

Dying To Be Me: My Journey from Cancer, to Near Death, to True Healing

It is a must read for anybody looking for some insight into life after death. There are several interviews on you tube where Anita shares her story.

Post Traumatic Stress Disorder; PTSD

"Post-Traumatic Stress Disorder (PTSD) is an anxiety disorder that may develop after exposure to a terrifying event or ordeal in which severe physical harm occurred or was threatened. Traumatic events that may trigger PTSD include violent personal assaults, natural or unnatural disasters, accidents, or military combat.[3].

PTSD was originally thought to only affect soldiers returning from a war zone however it has been expanded to include any individual suffering from unresolved trauma relating to intensely fear eliciting events.

This could be people living in a war zone, someone experiencing a natural disaster, the children of alcoholic or abusive parents, the spouse of a violent partner or the victim of a bullying or oppressive boss. The person relives the trauma in the form of flash backs or the trauma may be so deeply buried that the individual has only physical symptoms like chronic stress in the body : migraine headaches, backache, unexplained fatigue, digestive issues, chronically tight muscles that are unresponsive to stretching. He or she may be depressed or suffer anxiety. The individual may be hyper vigilant, always on guard. They may be extra sensitive to light, sound and crowds. PTSD affects people, physically, mentally and emotionally.

At the root of the trauma lies an unresolved reptilian brain response to the fear. Our Reptilian brain is our most primitive brain and it is responsible for the most basic functions that allow us to survive; heartbeat, body temperature and reflexes. One such primitive reflex governed by the reptilian brain is the startle reflex. If a baby gets a sudden fright it extends it limbs and recoils itself for protection. This reflex which responds to fear includes a program for body movement.

Having lived in war torn zones for many years trauma expert David Berceli discovered a number of phenomena regarding how the body reacts to stressful situations.

1: The body tends to curl up into the foetal position to protect itself.

2: It tends to discharge the stress through a tremor response or shaking.

He noticed many mammals in the wild do the exact same thing. If a dear is chased by a lion and escapes it undergoes a tremor or shaking period to return it to homeostasis. The event is then forgotten. The dear does not walk around mulling over the prospect of meeting a lion.

"The tremors are an organic response to the body being over excited. The tremor is actually a calming down of the body"

David Berceli PhD

The problem that Dr Berceli identified is that human's supress this natural reaction in order to save face or avoid humiliation in social settings.

You see our emotions have a vibrational quality that can be quantified on a scale. This was first done by David Hawkins in his book Power Versus Force.

The peak emotional states have a very high score like Love, Bliss and Peace. However the lower harmonic of emotions like Fear, Anger, Shame and Humiliation have very low scores. A low scoring emotion literally brings you down and a high scoring one literally uplifts you. The two lowest scores on the vibrational emotional ladder are humiliation and shame.

In order to avoid these extremely difficult emotions many people supress the body's natural response to fear inducing situations. So if you are being bullied by your peers as a young kid and it's very scary you may lock up the urge to shake or tremor to avoid humiliation. Unfortunately this locks the trauma up in your physical structure. How many times has a person hidden their natural fear response in a given lifetime? Certain individuals are way more sensitive to stressful situations and this might explain why only a certain percentage of the population is affected by PTSD.

What is the solution? There are many modalities available from the standard psychotherapy and drug rout to the more modern techniques like the emotional freedom technique. However what David Berceli discovered was that many people get stuck in a loop between their Limbic system which allows feelings to arise and their neo cortex which can comprehend and make sense of those feelings. Why?

The physical release that was required by the body via the nervous system never happened as the reptilian brain cannot be accessed by talk therapy.

The reptilian brain can however be accessed through movement. Dr Berceli developed a system called Trauma Release Exercises™ to create a means to physically release the effects of trauma. See http://www.bercelifoundation.org for further information and to locate a certified practitioner.

Chapter 11

Archetypes of the foundation

An archetype has been defined as:

"An original model or type after which other similar things are patterned; a prototype[1]"

In one way an archetype is like a personality type. In reality we are all a mix of a vast array of personalities. Sometimes these are called sub personalities or aspects of the self. At the highest levels of consciousness we realise that we are all One. This means that we have played all possible roles at one point or another. If not in this lifetime then in another. We have been Hero and Villain, Victim and Vanquisher.

"The whole world is a stage, and all the men and women merely actors. They have their exits and their entrances, and in his lifetime a man will play many parts, his life separated into seven acts. In the first act he is an infant, whimpering and puking in his nurse's arms. Then he's the whining schoolboy, with a book bag and a bright, young face, creeping like a snail unwillingly to school. Then he becomes a lover, huffing and puffing like a furnace as he writes sad poems about his mistress's eyebrows. In the fourth act, he's a soldier, full of foreign curses, with a beard like a panther, eager to defend his honour and quick to fight."

William Shakespeare

In looking at the different archetypes it is important not to judge any particular one right or wrong, good or bad. They all serve a purpose i.e. expand our consciousness and broaden our band-width of the human experience.

They enable us to love ourselves in all possible situations through all of the roles that we have played. All of these characters are all God's children seeking to be loved back to the oneness from whence they came.

Earth Mother

Our root chakra connects us to the earth. The earth is our Mother and she provides everything that our physical bodies require to sustain us. She also provides us with comfort and healing through her natural beauty and through her bounty of foods and herbal agents. When we are fully connected in to the earth through our root chakra we can receive all that we require to sustain our human experience. We are capable of nurturing ourselves. We can stand on our own two feet and take care of ourselves. We can provide for ourselves in terms of our material needs, food, clothing and shelter. We can provide for ourselves in terms of our mental and emotional needs. If we are not able, for whatever reason, to mother ourselves we may attempt to mother others in a bargaining quest to be mothered and loved in return . This is one of the forms of co-dependence.

The Co-dependant

I looked at co-dependency in chapter 10 on the behavioural aspects of the root chakra. If one does not have a direct line in to Mother earth via a strong and fully functional root chakra one looks for a power source outside of one's self. Everything is energy so if we don't get it in one way we can attract, generate or create it in other ways. The co-dependent tries to get energy from other persons, situations, behaviours or substances. The person with a weak root chakra may try to get energy from a relationship even if it is an abusive one. Violence towards a person is energy directed to them. It's very like the little kid who acts up just to get the attention of the parents. Even the parents screaming at him is better than being ignored. Co-dependency is a misdirected way of managing your energy field. There most likely will be some spiritual lessons thrown into the mix! The quicker one learns the spiritual lessons the quicker one can go back to the internal sourcing of energy.

The Warrior

Throughout our history as human beings we have had a belief that we need to fight to survive. Fight to defend our lands. Fight to defend our families. Fight to defend our basic rights. The warrior archetype will come up in your life when you go way beyond anger into the realm of rage and fury where for example you are willing to pummel someone to death in order to save your own life or the life of a loved one.

If we have been severely disrespected or dishonoured we may seek vengeance. We may be filled with a fire inside that's so strong it overtakes any rational thought process. This is a powerful force that can be drawn upon for self-preservation. If you are willing to embody the killing energy it is very unlikely that you will be attacked. It does not mean that you have to go there but the fact that you would be willing to creates a whole new dynamic in any particular altercation where your life might be threatened.

If you are always on the defensive, putting your barriers up, don't be surprised if your life is a constant battle field. When your defences are up you are operating from fear and fear is the energy that attracts attack and violence from others. A woman coming from a violent home will attract subsequent violent partners, as the fear and vibration of violence is still in her energy field. Until it is resolved she will attract persons with the same energetic vibration.

> "When I defend myself I am attacked"
>
> A Course in Miracles

Put the barriers down but be willing to kill and then you become the peaceful samurai: a guardian of the weak and a defender of peace.

The Victim

The victim always seems to be portrayed in a negative light. I suppose it's not surprising how that may be the case. The victim appears powerless and is full of self-doubt. He or she blames others for what's going wrong in their lives. But would a person who is living consciously ever play the victim? Is the victim an unconscious person playing out a role in order to gain consciousness? Is the victim playing a role for someone else in order to assist their soul's journey in some way?

Can you blame a child who is abused for being a victim of this abuse? Do you make that victimhood wrong? A child who has come from an abusive home clearly is a victim. Would you say to a 5 year old screaming in pain "Oh stop playing the victim"! I hope not! Is that appropriate to say to an adult who may be playing the role of the victim? What if part of their consciousness IS that 5 year old abused and abandoned child? Sometimes it's very appropriate to allow the person in question really act out the feelings and dialogue of the inner victim. This can be done in therapy or by exploring the roots of victimhood which for many lay in early childhood experiences.

The Inner Child

The inner child is a concept I came across many years ago while reading a book by a lady who has really inspired me greatly over the years, Gill Edwards, chartered clinical psychologist (since deceased). The book, Living Magically, was a catalyst for many new levels of awareness on my own journey.

Your inner child is that part of you that's fun loving, spontaneous and playful. There are however many other inner children. Many of them wounded. The wounded child is one who has suffered a hurt from the seemingly slight to the obviously grotesque. We all have wounded children that become trapped or frozen in time while they wait for our adult selves to rediscover them, hear their stories, allow them to vent their feelings and return them to wholeness again.

Exercise to meet your wounded child.

Sit with your spine upright, right up on your sits bones. Take a few deep belly breaths. Connect to the heavens through your crown chakra (the top of your head) and connect to the earth through your pelvic floor or root chakra. Imagine a column of pure white radiant light connecting you top to bottom connecting all the way through your heart chakra.

Continue the deep belly breaths and focus on your heart centre (I like to use the colours pink or green for this). Now take yourself back in time to an incident that caused your little self to be upset. What were you wearing? Where were you? What were you doing? What happened to upset you? Ask this little child what is wrong? Ask why they are upset and let them speak. Reassure them .Tell them you are listening and that you are right there for them. Tell them you are so sorry this happened. Say indignantly "this should never happen to a child, no child should have to experience this!" Ask them what they are feeling. Let them vent the emotion. If they are sad let them sit on your lap and cry. Wipe their tears and console them. If they are angry let them smash a pile of imaginary china plates. When I really wish to indulge an inner child I let them smash piles of the most expensive looking crystal. You are letting this child know they have the right to feel their feelings.

One of my own personal mini traumas was that I once visited my granny and she showed us these little baby chicks! I was so mesmerised by how cute and beautiful they were I wanted to bring one home! I was devastated when I was told I could not! The inner child does not like anything less than perfect love and perfect allowance for all of their needs no matter how bizarre we may think they are as adults. Every slight means "I am not loved"!!! In one of my visualisations I consoled my little child and this time she got to bring the baby chick home!

Some traumas of course are more severe and will need more time and possibly professional support.

"Coming to know and love the child within is not simply a light-hearted way of passing the odd half hour. It is an immensely powerful way of changing our lives"

  Gill Edwards, Living magically

There are many different types of inner child: happy, sad, disappointed, bored, abandoned, frightened, ashamed, guilt ridden, humiliated. We need to visit each one in turn to create more and more healing.

Spiritual adviser Matt Kahn advises that working on your inner child is one of the fastest ways to improve your prosperity. He states that if your inner child does not get the appropriate attention that he/she can be the saboteur extraordinaire of all of your efforts. Promise your inner child you will spend more time with him/her and not less to allow prosperity to come your way! The root chakra is the chakra of abundance and manifestation so if you are having difficulty with this area of your life this is a possible contributing factor.

Recreating your Inner Childs experience

Quantum Physics tells us there is only the present moment. Time is an illusion created by our minds. If this is the case then "time travel" is easy. You can travel "back" in time to visit your inner child and recreate any scenario you desire. Change the outcome of any situation that was stressful for your inner child.

You can even change your inner child's perspective of its parents. To do this journey inwards after centering yourself and breathing deeply a few times. Now ask your inner child to show you how it would have liked its mother to be using an animal to depict symbolically what he or she desired. Do the same with the father and ask your inner child to show you through animal symbolism which animal the child wanted. You can now imagine your inner child playing with animals. Being carried on the back of the animal or playing with it.

In shamanic traditions animal medicine is seen as very powerful. Each animal symbolises certain qualities and delivers a unique medicine for the human condition. This is an ancient tribal practice very appropriate for the root chakra.

The Bully

The Bully is another archetype connected to the root chakra. The bully is so unsure of how to stand in his or her own power that he or she tries to energetically rob the power of another person by pulling them out of alignment or knocking them off centre. You see if you stand firmly on your own two feet and maintain a strong root chakra you will have the strength to stand up for yourself and the bully is out of a job. The bully will try to suction energy off his /her prey by attaching energetic cords to the chakras of their victims. In the book Hands of Light, Physicist and Intuitive, Barbara Ann Brennan describes many methods that individuals use as an energetic defence system. In the case I will site she describes a bully (the archer) who gives cruel energetic blows to their prey:

"The archer unconsciously hopes this will cause enough pain to elicit anger, which will then give him an excuse to release his own anger in such a way as to avoid humiliation. In this wilful, precise, mental way, he tries to humiliate the other person and at the same time, avoid having feelings in the lower half of his body".

The lesson that the bully brings is to get his victim to stand up for him /herself. The lesson the bully needs to learn is also curiously the same, to stand on his or her own two feet and rely on their own connection to mother earth as a source of power rather than try to parasitically draw power from others.

Abuser

The bully above could be seen as an abuser. However there are other types of abusers to be considered from the most hideous in the form of child molestation, rape and domestic violence to more subtle forms of abuse we may unwittingly be subjecting ourselves to.

From that friend who is always asking you if you have put on a bit of weight , to that co-worker who is always making sarcastic comments about your work under the guise of humour to that girlfriend/boyfriend /spouse who polices your every move.

Sarcasm in many cases is a form of passive aggressive behaviour. It stems from a deep insecurity in the individual in question. The person usually has a lot of unresolved anger and is trying to channel it in a very dysfunctional way:

"If you want to be happier and improve your relationships, cut out sarcasm since sarcasm is actually hostility disguised as humour. Sarcasm is a subtle form of bullying and most bullies are angry, insecure, cowards. "

Clifford N. Lazarus, Ph.D. Clinical Psychologist

Sometimes abuse just involves one person. The abuser is you abusing yourself. This self-abuse could manifest in issues with food, drugs or even over exercising. People running themselves into the ground with too much exercise have serious safety and security issues that will not be resolved by relentless training. The abuse is hidden under a mask of discipline and dedication.

Stop and ask yourself "If I really felt safe would I be doing this?" or "What am I really afraid of here?" These questions could be applied to all of the archetypes identified in this section.

The Prostitute

We all know the classic form of prostitution; selling sex for money. However one can play the role of prostitute anytime one is willing to do something that dishonours the self. Are you stuck in a rut in a job that you hate? Are you in a relationship that's past its sell by date? Are you doing anything that is dishonouring you just to get a false sense of safety?

Remember all true safety comes from within. With Self Respect you gain the grace and ability to take actions that honour your Being. Be that leaving a job that's soul destroying or ending a relationship that is not nurturing you.

The sooner you feel safe in your body the sooner you can fire your inner prostitute. The fastest way to feel safe in your body is to practice relaxation techniques and the root chakra exercises in this book. Slowing your breathing is one of the quickest ways to relax your body.

The Reptile

The human brain can be divided into many different regions. The reptilian, the limbic or mammalian brain and the neocortex or neo mammalian brain. This was first identified by neuro scientist Paul MacLean.

The reptilian brain is our most primitive brain. It acts instantly, compulsively and is driven by the desire to be safe, the desire to find food, and the desire to find a mate. It's not rational but highly reactionary. Fear is its primary driver. The reptile in all of us comes into full force when anything threatens our safety or survival.

Examples of our inner reptile in action:

Making choices based on fear

Compulsivity

Reclusiveness

Reactionary

Reacting without consideration of the consequences

Reacting with no consideration of others

Feeling your actions are totally out of control

Explosive rage

The reptile is only concerned with his/her own survival. The more stressed a person is the more they retreat into their reptilian brains. So when you see a person building a bunker for the end of the world that is reptilian brain in full flight, when you see a person bolting down a meal at the end of a stressful day that is reptilian brain in action, when you see two women in a cat fight over a man or a man taking out another man who he thinks is eying his girlfriend up that is reptilian brain. These are all fear driven responses with no rational back up. So if you feel your inner reptile coming out, pause, take a deep breath and talk to it just like you would your inner child.

"Thank you my little reptile for watching my back but you know what all is well here. There's nothing to worry about!"

Have this conversation often to calm down your inner reptile. Make stress reduction a part of your daily routine so that you do not function solely from your reptile brain. Read the section on Post Traumatic Stress Disorder in chapter 10 to find out how to release deep reptilian trauma from past events.

The Miser

We all know that friend or acquaintance who never pays for anything. They are happy to receive gifts or be treated to lunch but rarely do they put their hand in their own pocket. We have an expression for this by labelling the person in question a "tight ass". The back side or buttocks are governed by the root chakra so the expression "tight ass" is very fitting. At the root of this issue lies the reptilian brained fear of safety and security. When the safety of the body is threatened one of the physiological responses in the human body is for all sphincter muscles to tighten up (a sphincter is a circular muscle that opens and closes like a valve). This is necessary to create enough spinal stability so the individual in question can fight or flee. The muscles of the rectum (your back passage) literally tighten up. The expression "tight ass" is not accidental! Your tight ass friend is actually living in fear and has some deep seated issues around money connected to survival.

The Addict

The addict could be a shopaholic, alcoholic, workaholic or sex addict to mention a few. Much of this is the search for a dopamine hit as a mechanism of yet again coping with a stress response. The addict does not feel safe to feel his or her real feelings. The addict in many ways is an inner child yanking at your sweater begging to be loved, received and comforted. Try some journeying towards your inner child and ask him/her what he/she really desires.

The Door Mat

The door mat is the quintessential people pleaser. This person is always looking for love and approval outside of themselves. If they were filled with Self Respect they would honour their own needs first. The door mat is so eager to please and make a good impression with others that they will say yes to requests without reviewing if that's what they would really like to do. In the end they have no time or space for themselves. They get very stressed and suffer from burnout.

The doormat essentially feels that their source of energy lies outside of themselves. Once they realise their source of energy is internal they won't have to reach out to others by people pleasing instead they can pause and assess whether any interaction is truly heart felt or an attempt to get praise or respect from others. The doormat needs to learn appropriate interpersonal boundaries. What behaviour is acceptable from others and what is not? Learning to say no is one of the most difficult aspects especially for women. We have been socially conditioned to say yes to everything and anything and in the end this builds resentment and exhaustion.

Exercises:

Make a list of the behaviours that are unacceptable to you.

Pause, take a breath and let somebody know how you feel calmly if they do or say something unacceptable.

Use expressions like "I'll think about it" or "I'll sleep on it" before agreeing to do anything for anybody else.

Learn to put your own needs and desires first. If something makes you feel heavy it's not in your best interest. If it makes you feel light then it will be a contribution to you and your life.

The Interdependent

The interdependent person has arrived at a state of balance and wholeness within themselves. They are independent in so far as they know they are capable of doing everything themselves however they also love themselves enough to allow others to offer, help , assistance, support and contribution to their lives. They have arrived at a state of discernment whereby they can identify the individuals that are truly a contribution to their wellbeing and overall sense of happiness. The relationship of the interdependent person with themselves is still the number 1 priority in their lives. All other relationships in this person's life are simply a reflection of their own self-love. When the interdependent person has a relationship it is one of equality. Both people grow and expand from the process of interacting.

A co-dependent relationship is on the other hand a one way street; one person gives and the other person takes.

One person feels a temporary uplift and the other person feels drained. With interdependent relationships both people come away feeling uplifted. There is no sense of debt or owing or what I call "investment banking love" whereby you are looking for a return on your caring.

The interdependent person is neither co-dependent or overly independent. He or she can move seamlessly between spending time on their own or interacting with others.

I learned a valuable aspect of this lesson on a Connemara mountain side. I was walking down the mountain after trekking up with a group of people. I had not been hiking in several years. The descent was fairly tricky since it was very wet and boggy in places. One of the guys on the trip reached his hand out to assist me on a few occasions and I rebuffed him. I thought to myself, "I have got this covered; I can do this on my own". A few feet later the ground went from under me as I fell into a big hole, got the fright of my life and slammed my right side really bad. My knee was throbbing. I got a surge of adrenaline and just managed to make it down the rest of the way. Later on I asked my body what it was trying to tell me. A few hours later I got the reply "Clare, you are trying to be too independent, it's ok to get help and assistance from time to time. It does not mean you are lazy or incapable."

The right side of your body is your action taking side, your doing side and your independence side. You can have too much of a good thing! The left side of your body is your receiving side, your ability to be nurtured and your ability to be vulnerable. Life is a dance between both sides. Overuse of one side or underuse of the other leads to the dysfunctional states of co-dependency or neediness on the one hand or over independence and isolation on the other.

So "doing the leg work" is you taking action, and "getting a leg up" is the ability to receive help and assistance from friends. If you have the discernment to know which leg to work from in any given moment you will be successful in any endeavour.

Chapter 12

Health conditions and Diseases of the foundation

Lack of functional strength

Every person on the planet requires a minimum standard of strength to carry out the activities of daily living. Something as simple as getting up off the sofa can become an impossibility for some elderly people and this can be incapacitating and soul destroying. Simple things like being able to carry your luggage not only makes you independent it also protects your body biomechanically. Being strong is the number 2 predictor of your lifespan.

The solution to this dilemma of poor functional strength is to start a weight training program. Beginners may start with body weight exercises and then progress on to dumbbell and barbell work. It is advisable to get instruction to make sure you are doing the exercises safely, effectively and progressively. One achieves a very basic level of functional strength from activities like Pilates and yoga, however to develop the level of strength that's life extending then weight training is key.

Muscle wasting/sarcopenia

Sarcopenia is the degenerative loss of muscle tissue that can occur as we age due to lack of appropriate exercise. The maintenance of lean body mass (your lean body mass is the tissue that is left once the fat is removed) is the number one predictor of your life span. Progressive weight training is the single best method to preserve and build muscle tissue. It needs to be accompanied by appropriate nutrition to assist the muscle building process.

Biomechanical Dysfunctions

Biomechanics as it pertains to the body is the science of muscle and joint function. Without healthy biomechanics the body breaks down. Symptoms like low back pain, joint pain and injuries are all addressed under this topic.

Modern living is very conducive to persons developing biomechanical disorders. Low back pain and dysfunction is epidemic in the western world. It's estimated that at least 80% of the population will complain of low back pain or weakness at some stage in their lives[1].

Many individuals end up getting a hip replacement as early as age 50.

The cause of many biomechanical issues is wide and varied from:

- Ergonomics at the work place. If you are seated for long periods of time this sets the stage for muscle imbalance and weakness.
- Lack of exercise or inappropriate exercise.
- Over use. Doing too much or too many repetitive patterns can cause imbalances.
- Not enough recovery relative to your training.
- Not enough stretching or over stretching the wrong muscles.
- Poor "software programing" with regards to the bodies strategy for movement and stabilisation.
- Internal organ stress causing a dysfunction of muscle groups on the same nerve path ways.

Sometimes muscles are weak not in and of themselves but because the signals from the nerves serving them is weak. An under-functioning or stressed internal organ can therefore neurologically rob a given muscle of its appropriate nerve signalling. This is called visceral-somato reflex. So having indigestion could actually contribute to or cause back pain!

What is the solution? I always recommend that everybody get a thorough biomechanical assessment to get an understanding of which muscles need to be stretched and which need to be strengthened in an integrative way. Stretching in isolation without strengthening is meaningless and may make certain conditions worse. To find a coach who can assess you properly and design appropriate training programs see www.chekinstitute.com. For advanced trainees who already have excellent stability and biomechanical balance find a trainer at www.poliquingroup.com

Arthritis

Arthritis is a type of joint pain caused by inflammation. There are over 100 types of arthritis. A diet promoting lower inflammation will greatly assist. The anti-inflammatory nutrients listed in the supplements chapter may greatly assist however individualisation of one's diet is key. Metabolic typing would be a great starting point and in addition I would recommend a food sensitivity test. Once you find out the foods you may be reacting to you can remove them. This calms the immune system and reduces inflammation.

Some individuals have found relief by removing the Nightshade family of vegetables from their diet. These include potatoes, tomatoes, varieties of peppers, eggplant or aubergine and goji berries. Others have found relief by eating a low purine diet. Foods rich in purines include: anchovies, sardines, all offal like liver and kidney and many varieties of meat.

This approach is all part and parcel of learning Self Care which is the bed rock of health and wellness generation.

On an energetic level diseases can be messages from your body as it demands your attention to treat it in a loving way. They can also be your bodies way of communicating to you emotional disturbance that you have locked away in your body unresolved.

Let's break the energetics down:

Inflammation: the fire inside, unexpressed anger turns to a rage and fury that cannot be expressed by the individual and so the anger and its close cousin resentment are turned inward.

Joints: That which supports us and holds us up in life. For many people our support network is our family. If we don't feel supported by our loved ones we get angry and resentful. Sometimes the individual is the one giving all the support but they don't receive any themselves and this builds resentment. The person can then become bitter and twisted just like their joints.

Movement: Unresolved emotions cripple us and stop us from moving forward in life. Remember you have to be fully present in your body to feel your feelings. When you are not present in your body the back log catalogue builds and builds and so rage and fury are the end result of anger which has been bottled up over a lifetime. If you can't feel or express anger, then the rage and fury which is even more intense, will be almost impossible for you to acknowledge let alone express. Persons who have made anger, rage, fury and hate wrong in their universe do not give themselves permission to own and express these energetic vibrations. Remember all they represent is a different quality of energetic vibration. Our judgement of them as bad or wrong or evil locks them into our bodies, and our bodies which do not judge, simply relay the truth of our feelings back to us.

So what is the solution? I would recommend a strength training program using weights. Research from Tufts University has shown a reduction in pain symptoms of 43% over a course of 16 weeks of weight training intervention in subjects with osteoarthritis [2].

Individualisation of the training program is the key so as not to exacerbate any existing areas that are particularly stressed.

Pilate's studio based training which uses a range of spring resistance equipment has also proved very popular with arthritis sufferers:

"Clinical Pilate's exercises have shown positive effects on decreasing the pain, improving function and general health perception. Clinical Pilates Exercises can be considered as reliable exercise model in children with Juvenile Idiopathic Arthritis. [3]"

Once you are exercising get some individualised guidance on your nutrition. Perhaps explore metabolic typing or getting a food sensitivity test done.

Start the process of getting in touch with deep feelings that you may have unwittingly buried. Give yourself permission to honour every feeling that comes up. Journaling can help here, also things like counselling or art therapy. Is your inner child bucking mad? Chances are high! Why not try some inner journeying to your inner child to see what he or she may be fuming mad about!

Because every single person on the planet is unique there is no singular approach for a disease process. A lot of the time it's a process of personal investigation that may be assisted by some outside intervention like testing. In most cases a disease process is a call to look within.

Inflammation

Inflammation is not a disease but a natural phenomenon in the body. Acute inflammation initiates a repair response in the body. If you stub your toe it gets red and swollen. This is an example of inflammation in action. There is another type of inflammation that is silent and chronic. This is the body's reaction to other types of assault that the body may be exposed to daily. It's this type of low grade chronic inflammation that becomes the bed rock of many of the diseases of modern man. These diseases include Arthritis, Diabetes, Heart disease, Alzheimer's , Pain, Obesity, Food sensitivities, Acne, Irritable bowel disease, Hashimotos Thyroiditis, Fibromyalgia, Lupus and even Cancer.

Inflammation is mediated by compounds known as cytokines. Cytokines are basically cell signallers or communicators between cells. There are many different varieties of cytokines and they are very involved in all immune response, inflammatory reactions and trauma response.

In a healthy person inflammation is a natural and temporary reaction to a perceived threat on the body or an injury. That threat could come in the form of a food the body thinks is an invader, a pathogen in the form of a bacterium or virus or other disease causing agent, a toxin, a stressor in the form of a mental or emotional trauma. Inflammation in theory, then, brings the body back to homeostasis or balance again. The problem with modern living, especially Western Living, is that there is more or less always something to compromise your health.

 That processed breakfast cereal you ate for breakfast, the traffic fumes you inhaled on your way to work, the stress coursing through your veins as you try to meet the next deadline, the emotional toxicity as you try to deal with the work place bully, the pathogen you unwittingly picked up at the work canteen buffet all keep you in a perpetual state of inflammation. When that inflammation is let run relentlessly the bedrock for the killer diseases of our time are sown.

So how do you know if you have high levels of inflammation? Well for starters if you have any of the diseases listed above then you are highly inflamed. If you are packing fat around your waistline you are highly inflamed. If you have elevated cholesterol (especially the LDL and VLDL) you are highly inflamed. If you have a high body fat percentage even if you are a normal weight you are highly inflamed. If you suffer with food sensitivities you are highly inflamed. If you suffer with stiff aching joints you are highly inflamed. If you over-train your body you are highly inflamed. If you get a lot of fluid retention you are highly inflamed.

There are many tests for inflammation including High Sensitivity C-reactive protein, Homocysteine, Fibrinogen, Tumour necrosis factor alpha, Interleukin 1 beta, interleukin 6 and interleukin 8.

So what do you do if you suspect you are very inflamed or you have had tests done that confirm high levels of inflammation?

1. Find out which foods are raising inflammation levels in your body. Get a sensitivity test done.

2. Get to bed on time and get a good night's sleep. People with sleep disturbance have higher levels of inflammation.

3. Optimise your body composition through a healthy individualised diet incorporating resistance exercise.

4. Avoid over training and excessive aerobic exercise. A 2006 study of 60 participants of the 2004 and 2005 Boston Marathons, found decreased right ventricular systolic function in the runners,(a measure of heart function) caused by an increase in inflammation and a decrease in blood flow[4].

Also Dr. Arthur Siegel, director of Internal Medicine at Harvard's McLean Hospital, has found that long distance running is correlated with high levels of inflammation which may increase incidences of cardiac events[5].

5. Avoid being a couch potato. Moderate exercise has been shown to reduce inflammation.

6. Introduce some anti-inflammatory foods to your diet like cherries, turmeric, chilli peppers, garlic, acerola juice, and wild salmon. Just make sure you do not have sensitivity to these foods.

7. Develop supportive relationships. A recent study has shown that social rejection leads to increases in inflammatory markers[6].

8. Make friends with your inner rage! Vent it during an intense weight training session. Boxing and contact martial arts can also be excellent to purge this deep supressed emotion.

9. Avoid foods that promote the formation of Advanced Glycation End products (AGES). AGEs are protein molecules that have essentially become caramelised by sugar. This means the molecule is totally damaged and disease causing. Foods that form AGEs are sugars and foods that turn into sugar like bread, pasta and cereal grains. Highly refined and processed sugars are the worst offenders. A

RAGE is a receptor for an Advanced Glycation End product. This receptor is hypothesised to have a causative effect in a range of inflammatory diseases such as diabetic complications and heart disease. Its these AGEs that damage skin and cause wrinkles :

"As AGEs accumulate, they damage adjacent proteins in a domino-like fashion," explains dermatologist Fredric Brandt, MD.

10. Get your ratio of omega 6 to omega 3 fats right. Too many omega 6 fats (largely found in vegetable oils and nuts) are pro inflammatory. Omega 3 fats are anti-inflammatory. Modern man has a ratio of 20; 1 or even 50; 1 of omega 6 to omega 3 fatty acids. This is a disaster. The cave man was speculated to have had a one to one ratio. Whatever way you slice it you need to get those vegetable oils out! No more sunflower or canola oil for you! Take a fish oil supplement as recommended in the supplements chapter. A teaspoon of pure refined fish oil per day works for most.

Fatigue

Your vitality and energy levels come from your root chakra. Fatigue is the number one reason that people report to their Doctors office. There are multiple contributing factors however this is a basic check list:

1. Are you exercising too little or too much? 3 times a week would be a minimum recommendation for most. Huge volumes of training like triathlon may be draining your body's ability to recover.

2. Quantity and quality of sleep. Most people require 7-8 hours' sleep. Quality of sleep means you don't wake up. If you are deficient in key nutrients (see next step) this can cause sleep disturbance.

3. Nutrient deficiency. If you are missing out or low on some key nutrients be they B vitamins or iron or a host of others then your energy will be low. The best bet is to get some comprehensive blood work done to assess your overall nutrient profile. Otherwise you are just guessing.

4. You are suffering from "burn out". Some people call this adrenal fatigue however it's much more complex. The adrenals are part of the Hypothalamus, Pituitary and Adrenal axis and as such the adrenals themselves are a "down-stream" organ. A useful test to get done is an adrenal stress index where your cortisol rhythm is tested. Some companies also do DHEA. This gives an idea of how well your body is adapting to stress and if your energy production rhythm (circadian rhythm) is healthy.

5. Too much time indoors and not enough time in Nature. If you are inside in a stuffy office all day and remain indoors when you go home you will not get enough exposure to fresh air and sunlight and Nature exposure which is vital to your human organism. Make time to get outdoors every day.

6. Eating the wrong nutritional plan for your body. Certain people do well on low fat diets, others do better low carb and others still are a mix between the two. If you don't fine tune your body's nutritional needs you will not get efficient energy

production. Metabolic typing is an excellent start to find the right fuel mix for you.

Go to http://www.mt-advisors.info/ to find an advisor in your area. Alternately many (including myself!) give consults on line.

7. Poor digestion means you are not getting access to the nutrients in your food. The major disruptor of digestion is stress. Follow the stress reduction techniques in this book to optimise your digestion.

8. Lack of balance in overall lifestyle. All work and no play makes Jack a dull boy or so the saying goes. Well all work and no play makes Jack a very tired boy too! What are you doing for fun, for relaxation, for creativity, for nature time, spiritual time and social time? If your life is polarised to only focus on one or two areas don't be surprised if you're tired. Identify areas that need a boost and start prioritising your time to include areas you have neglected.

9. One or more relationships in your life are draining you. Is it your partner, co-worker, friend, Mother or boss? Ask the question: who or what is draining my energy? Negative people who constantly complain are energy vampires. Make yourself the number one priority in your life and cut ties with the drainers and complainers. Your vitality will increase instantly!

10. All of the grounding exercises in this book and the root chakra bio-energetic exercises all boost energy long term. If you are very tired this style of exercise may be more appropriate than very intense training at least till you have replenished your body's chi or life force.

Trainers, Drainers and Complainers

One of the things that influences your energy far more than exercise, sleep, nutrition or vitamins is the company you keep. So in this next section, I am going to look at the trainers, drainers and complainers keeping you fat, weak, sick and tired.

Trainers

Christiaan Huygens, a Dutch mathematician and scientist, and the inventor of the pendulum clock, was the first person to observe a phenomenon called "Coupled Oscillations". Basically when two pendulums that were swinging out of sync were brought near each other they started to swing in sync. This is a process that has been called **entrainment.**

This is observed in the inanimate world of physics, however in biological systems similar entrainment patterns can be observed. Women who live together in close proximity for several months find their menstrual cycles becoming synchronised, a phenomenon known as the McClintock effect[7].

Basically the people we hang out with most frequently have the potential to entrain us to their vibration, be that habit, way of thinking, beliefs, or behaviours. This can work for us or against us depending on our level of awareness. If we hang out with proactive, inspiring and energising people this can have an expansive uplifting effect in our lives. If we hang out with the drainers and complainers of the world it can have the opposite effect unless we are masters of maintaining a high vibrational state in our energy fields.

Drainers and Complainers

The drainers and complainers of the world are in vast supply. These people have been described as energy vampires, energy sponges and energy parasites. They literally try to suck the life force out of you. You will know you are around one if you were in a good mood and all of a sudden your energy and mood tanks. These people are always focusing and talking about what is wrong in their lives and why everyone else is wrong and bad. The "Haters" on the internet are a classic example of this phenomenon.

The drainers and complainers of the world are not masters of their energy field and so they seek to sabotage the energy of others. Drainers and complainers have no interest in stepping it up and taking responsibility for their lives. Their default mode is to blame, criticise, defer, procrastinate and make excuses why they can't do X, Y, Z. The way you can identify these people most easily is if you hear the phrase **"I HAVE NO CHOICE"**

Now there is a critically important difference between a person who is stepping into their vulnerability (an advanced stage of Self Mastery) and a complainer or drainer. The vulnerable person speaks their truth (in the appropriate setting with a trusted friend or therapist) as part of a process of being brutally honest with themselves without judgement, blame or expectation. They are very proactive in taking the appropriate steps to rectify their situation. They take action and responsibility to change their circumstances.

The drainers and complainers have no intention to change! Why should they! They are too busy robbing your energy bank account. They piss and they moan and complain just to get your attention and energy. You can recognise these people probably most easily by their lack of willingness to do anything proactive despite being offered help or professional advice.

I remember I had a client one time many years ago who was willing to do everything except the one thing she needed to do to lose the weight. She needed to really focus on detoxification. Any time I brought up the subject she was either too busy, it wasn't a good time, she had …..Wait for it….**NO CHOICE.** Needless to say this client was getting far more mileage pissing and moaning to me about her body woes than actually doing the one thing that would have transformed her, i.e. stepping into her power and doing what needed to be done. I ended up firing this client as she was a constant drain on my energy. Then I made space for clients who were ready to follow through on my advice.

The fastest way to lose weight

Take an inventory of all the drainers and complainers in your life. Are they really enhancing your life and adding to it or are they a mill stone around your neck?

Eliminate them from your life or reduce your time with them substantially.

Do not entertain their whinging.

I was travelling back from a Pilates Workshop in London on one occasion and somebody had taken my seat without asking. I wasn't bothered as it was only a short flight so I let it go. The guy in question who was severely obese and clearly very physiologically stressed started to piss and moan about how the airline was always late and crap (they are in fact 90% on time and we landed on time!!)

He tried to "hook into my energy field" so I promptly put on my head phones to listen to a really great radio show I had recorded with a kick ass powerful and proactive presenter. I could feel the guy seething as he was looking for somebody to explode on! That day it was not going to be me! Yippee! Eventually he gave one of the staff, an innocent bystander, an earful.

The drainers and complainers feed on your attention as they are not attuned to their own personal power. You know when you are at the zoo and you see a sign:

"DO NOT FEED THE ANIMALS"

Do not feed the drainers and complainers of life with your attention and try to remember the difference between vulnerability and complaining.

I avoided gaining 250lbs of toxic weight on my London flight as I was not willing to play catch the poo ball with this guy!!

How much of your excess weight and/or exhaustion is a protection/effect from the drainers and complainers of the world?

Chronic Muscle Tension

Many times I see in my client's chronic tension in the muscles creating severe flexibility restrictions and bodies that only know how to generate force from the shoulder girdle up. In Chinese medicine there are two energy currents; an upward one taking us up to the heavens or our mental space and a downward one connecting us to the earth and our bodies.

Too much living in the head takes us out of the body and drives all energy upwards. This leads to shoulder girdle tension, neck pain, scalp tension and locked up hips.

When you are relaxed your facial muscles relax, your jaw relaxes, the root of your tongue relaxes, the crease between your eyebrows relaxes, your brow unfurrows, your shoulders drop and you can feel yourself anchored in your legs and body. You can feel both feet on the ground. This feels very relaxing.

Mind body disciplines like Pilates, yoga and Tai Chi and Chi Gung can be very helpful to achieve this state as can the bioenergetic exercises in this book which channel the energy current downward to your root chakra.

Other ways to cope with chronic muscle tension:

1. Get biomechanically assessed and get your trainer to design a stretch program for you that's customised to your own bodies restrictions. This will work way more effectively than a generic routine. Stretching long weak muscles only generates a greater fear response in the body as it makes you more unstable. Look up a trainer at www.chekinstitute.com

2. Get a good deep tissue massage from a specialist. Aromatherapy massage can also be highly effective due to the healing qualities of scent. Your sense of smell is a root chakra phenomenon.

3. Massage yourself regularly with relaxing oils like lavender or rose. Self-massage is a key component of Ayurvedic medicine and is an excellent self-care exercise.

4. Try a hot bath with a few cups of dissolved Epsom salts. The magnesium content seeps into the body generating relaxation of your muscles.

5. Try meditation. It could be as simple as observing your breath and slowing it down. When you slow your breath your body relaxes. Guided meditation is also possible. Whatever you do find a practice that works for you and that you can commit to.

6. Sauna therapy. This can be very relaxing for tight muscles especially if the sauna is the Infra-red kind. Infra-red rays penetrate the muscles at a deeper level relieving stress and tension.

7. Hydrotherapy. If you go into a spa or pool with specialised water jets that you can direct at your muscles this can be amazing release. It's one of my personal favourites. Couple with a sauna and its tension release heaven! When I lived in Germany for many years this was an almost weekly ritual.

8. Foam Rolling. You can purchase a foam roller online or in most sporting goods stores. You can use these to roll out tight muscles. Start with a softer roller before moving to a firmer one.

9. Acupuncture can also release a lot of stress out of the body. Remember if an internal organ is under stress it can reflex to a given muscle group making it weak and/or chronically tense.

10. Try stress relieving nutrients suggested in the supplements chapter.

11. Try progressive muscular relaxation:

Example:

Lay on the ground on an exercise mat on your back. Start by tensing one foot for 5-10 seconds. Scrunch it up! Then completely relax for 10 s. Now do the calf of the same leg. Tighten for 5-10 seconds and then relax for 10 seconds. Progress to front of the thigh then right butt cheek. Then do the other leg. Now do both butt cheeks together. Now follow up with abs, chest, biceps and fists. Now hunch your shoulders up and really relax down. Now tighten your face and relax. Clench your teeth and relax. It's important not to hurt or strain yourself while generating the tension. You want to teach your body the difference between contraction and relaxation. The more you practice the better you get at isolating the muscular contractions to a given region.

Constipation/ Diarrhoea

The large intestine is the most earth based internal organ. It literally connects us to the earth. When functioning optimally this is the region where a lot of water is reabsorbed into the body and the stool or bowel movement is formed. Some salts are also reabsorbed here and trillions of bacteria ferment the colon contents and generate some vitamins and assist our immunity and health in ways that we are only beginning to understand.

When the colon is not functioning in a healthy way one of two things happens. We either get constipated or our bowel movement becomes too loose watery and frequent which is known as diarrhoea.

There are many theories as to what constitutes constipation. However my standard is that I like to see people having a bowel movement daily. In native cultures where there is almost no colon cancer as an example the typical transit time of the colon is between 12 and 24 hours. The colon transit time is defined as the length of time it takes for the food to be excreted from your body from the time of ingestion.

Discovering your own transit time:

Eat **either** a good serving of red beets or take 6-7 charcoal tablets which will cause your bowel movement to have a distinctive colour. (red in case of the beets and black in case of the charcoal). Now take note of the date and time you did this. Now take note when the substance you ingested reappears in your stools. Note the date and time. From the above data you should be able to calculate your transit time. Anything greater than 24 hours and you can consider yourself constipated.

What to do if you are constipated:

1. Start to drink more water. Most people need about 39 ml per Kg of body weight (or 0.6-0.7 ounces of water per lb of body weight) daily. You may need more if you are sweating a lot due to intense exercise or living in a hot or humid climate. You may need less if you are substituting your diet with electrolytes.

2. Get plenty of fibrous vegetables and fruits in your diet. Things like broccoli, Brussels sprouts, artichokes, raspberries, pears and avocados give a great source of fibre.

3. Check your magnesium levels. As much as 70% of westerners are deficient in this vital macro mineral. Start taking a supplement of an amino acid chelated form (magnesium citrate or malate or fumarate or glycinate). Start with 400-500mg in the evening. You may need more and a red blood cell magnesium test will show the degree of your deficiency. If you take too much you will get loose stools. Spread the magnesium out over the last few meals and snacks of the day for best absorption.

4. Try the stress reduction techniques in this book. The vast majority of clients I see with constipation are highly stressed. Remember when you are stressed the sphincter muscles of the body tighten up in preparation for fight or flight. That means your anal sphincter tightens up! It needs to completely relax to have a bowel movement.

5. Start exercising the body through full range of motion. The natural peristaltic wave motion along

the entire gastro-intestinal tract is enhanced by exercising the body particularly in ways where the body must generate intra-abdominal pressure. Peristalsis is the natural muscular contraction that happens along the gut wall. Deep squats are a fantastic example of the type of exercise that helps. Even body weight ones will help.

6. Consider adding an additional fibre supplement e.g. ground flaxseeds, psyllium or glucomannon. These are all gluten free for those with a sensitivity.

What to do if you have diarrhoea:

1. If it's a regular occurrence or you have been diagnosed with irritable bowel syndrome get your doctor or health care provider to order a stool test to identify any pathogens that may be causing the problem. These can then be targeted specifically.

2. Get a food sensitivity test done. This will greatly reduce inflammation in the body which can drive this type of response.

3. Avoid foods you know are particularly hard for you to digest. Raw foods are a disaster for many with this issue. Even raw juices can trigger the problem. Beans and legumes can also be notoriously difficult to digest. Use a food diary to keep track of your symptoms.

4. Chronic ongoing stress or past unresolved mental or emotional stress can be a huge driver in cases of irritable bowel. Many of my clients see symptoms flare up if they are going through a stressful period in their lives. Stress management is therefore a critical element in an overall approach.

5. Get tested to see how balanced your gut flora are. You will have to go to a doctor or specialist to order a test for you.

"Small intestinal bacterial overgrowth is associated with irritable bowel syndrome. Eradication of the overgrowth eliminates irritable syndrome by study criteria in 48% of subjects"[8].

6. Consider taking a good quality probiotic

The strains Lactobacillus acidophilus NCFM and Bifidobacterium lactis BI-07 have shown favour in the research for IBS patients[9].

And in another study:

Probiotic bacteria Lactobacillus acidophilus NCFM and Bifidobacterium lactis Bi-07 were shown to reduce symptoms of functional bowel disorders [10].

Colitis and other disorders of the Colon

Colitis is an inflammation of the colon so all of the suggestions that applied to the diarrhoea section will also apply to this profile.

If the transit time of the colon is too slow then the body can become auto-intoxicated by reabsorbing toxins into the system. Some naturopaths believe this is one possible contributory factor to Colon Cancer.

If the transit time of the colon is too fast then not enough nutrients will have been absorbed in the small intestine leading to malnourishment.

The Colon represents how in flow and in tune we are with the natural rhythms of life. All fear responses can either give us constipation or diarrhoea. The expression "Scared shitless" is perhaps a less than eloquent but telling metaphor for how our emotional state creates effects in the body.

When a client is constipated I also ask the question "What are you not willing to let go of?" If we hold on to resentment or we are control freaks of the universe don't be surprised if constipation shows up.

On one of my first visits to my brother who lives in the United States I asked him why do the Americans call the toilet the "Rest Room"? His reply? "Well you're not going to get much more relaxed than when you use the toilet."

So relax more, go with the flow, stop holding onto resentment and fear and see how happy your colon could be.

Frequent Urination

Frequent urination is having to go to the bathroom more than 8 times a day. Many things can drive it like prostate cancer, diabetes, being pregnant, infections, cystitis or certain neurological disturbances. The first port of call is to rule all of these issues out by visiting your Doctor or Urologist. If the disturbance continues the following can be considered.

Your pelvic floor may be very weak and require some strengthening. The Pelvic Floor Exercises given in chapter 5 will help here. Pilates exercises are one of the best methods to rewire the functioning of the pelvic floor. The pelvic floor function is intimately connected with breathing mechanics and functioning of other muscles of the abdominal wall such as the transversus abdominus (the muscle use to pull your belly button in). Pilates is one of the best methods to re-educate the software programing of this co-ordination.

Once the pelvic floor is "firing" correctly you can get it really strong with loaded squats and deadlifts however there is an endurance component to the pelvic floor that is best trained during an hour long Pilates class for example. In a recent study on strengthening the pelvic floor Pilates exercise was compared to standard medical pelvic floor training.

Lead study author Dr Patrick Culligan, MD said

""The Pilates group received all the pelvic-floor benefits enjoyed by the PFMT (pelvic-floor muscle training) group, but they also received [the] full-body benefits of Pilates as well.[11]"

Another driver of frequent urination is fear and anxiety. Try the stress reduction techniques in this book with some pelvic floor strengthening and see how you get on.

Stress Urinary Incontinence.

Incontinence is an inability to maintain control of your bladder. If you have complete incontinence you have to be surgically fitted with an incontinency bag. Not very nice and unfortunate for some who have this condition. This is the worst case scenario. There are many cases however where people become temporarily incontinent due to a stressor. Somebody makes you laugh uncontrollably, you sneeze, you lift a heavy suitcase out of your car and all of a sudden you have a leakage of your bladder. Not the kind of thing you want to chat to friends about over lunch, right? It's an embarrassing situation but way more common than most people realise. Here are some of the statistics:

It affects an estimated 15 million women in the United States alone.

It affects 17% of men and women aged 30-39 and 29% of the 60-70 age group.

Approximately, 1 out of 3 women over the age of 45, and 1 out of every 2 women over 65 have stress urinary incontinence.

In approximately 20% of men who have had prostate surgery some degree of stress incontiance will continue to be a significant problem one year post-surgery

Source of statistics: The National Association for Continence

www.nafc.org

Over the years I have had many clients, particularly female clients with this issue. Deconditioned clients who have not exercised for a long time are very susceptible as are the overweight and those who are pregnant or have had children and omitted a post pregnancy pelvic floor reconditioning practice. Sedentary work is also a huge contributor.

The muscles of the pelvic floor are designed to not only control your bladder they are designed to hold all of your internal organs in place and help generate intra-abdominal pressure to stabilise the spine. In the clients I have had with weak pelvic floor and stress incontinence they always had a weak back and or back pain on initial assessment.

In fact stress incontinence is one of the first warning signs that your low back is vulnerable to injury.

What is the solution? As with the urinary frequency issue start off with the pelvic floor exercises in chapter 5 of this book. Progress on to do Pilates classes, group or private and then integrate into a weight training routine.

Remember the body has to relearn how to "fire" the muscles of the pelvic floor and integrate them with correct breathing and abdominal wall function. We move from isolated exercises for the pelvic floor to integrated ones. You may be able to contract your pelvic floor on its own fairly easily but making sure it's still working in an integrated way with an explosive and loaded exercise like a kettle bell swing its several levels above in difficulty. The progression to recovery is as follows:

Isolated pelvic floor exercises, integrated Pilates exercises, weight training, explosive or power training e.g. Olympic lifts, Kettle Bell Swings.

Low Libido, Erectile Dysfunction and Sex addiction.

Any scenario whereby a person totally closes off their sexual desires or has their life completely ruled by them as is the case with sex addiction is an example of yet another dysfunction of the root chakra.

There can be mechanical contributory factors, biochemical ones with neurotransmitters and hormones and psychological ones.

Let's take erectile dysfunction as an example. It may be a simple mechanical issue of poor blood flow due to arteriosclerosis. It could be driven by decline of sex hormones like testosterone or it could be brought on by psychogenic reasons like anxiety.

What is the solution to these issues?

Get a complete physical examination to rule out any issues of this nature. Get biomechanically healthy so that your pelvic girdle is stable and your pelvic floor is optimally functioning.

Build up to some vigorous weight training 2-4 times per week. Heavy lifting stimulates testosterone production.

Many people notice their sex drive go up with weight training!

Get rid of any excess weight especially excess body fat. This impairs testosterone production.

When you are in shape your confidence goes up. I call testosterone the hormone of confidence. Boost your confidence and it may just boost your testosterone. Boost your testosterone and it may just boost your confidence. I have seen this many times in the weight room especially with females. When your confidence goes up you can in the words of Justin Timberlake "bring sexy back"!

Sex addiction is like all other addictions. There are biochemical components linked to dopamine, serotonin and the sex hormones themselves. Getting these markers tested by your Doctor would be a great start. According to addiction specialist Gabor Mate all addictions are simply a mechanism to avoid feeling our emotional pain. Counselling and support group work for many is essential.

Osteoporosis

Osteoporosis is also known as brittle bone disease. People who have it have a lower bone density than desirable. Due to this low bone density persons afflicted are susceptible to fractures at the slightest impact.

Many people are aware of the importance of calcium in the bone building process however most people with osteoporosis are not in fact deficient in calcium. Osteoporosis is most common in females but its rates are rising also in males.

The process of building bone is a very complex one and like many systems in the body it's a delicate balance of a two sided process; the bone building of the osteoblasts and the bone dissolving of the osteoclasts.

Key vitamins and minerals in the bone building process:

The body clearly requires calcium to build bones however many other nutrients work in concert to establish bone density.

These include:

-Vitamin D to help with calcium absorption. Worldwide an estimated 1 billion people have inadequate levels of vitamin D in their blood[12].

- Magnesium which converts vitamin D into its active form (many women diagnosed with osteoporosis have low levels of magnesium).

-Zinc which enhances vitamin D function and is a co factor for alkaline phosphatase an enzyme very important in bone formation. Zinc deficiency is becoming more prevalent worldwide.

Boron, Silicon and Vitamin K are also key players in bone building.

If you are missing out on any one of these nutrients your bone building may be compromised.

Healthy levels of oestrogen and testosterone are required for bone formation.

High levels of inflammation impair bone formation.

Poor blood sugar regulation impacts bone formation in a negative way as do AGEs or advanced glycation end products.

If you have high levels of a substance known as sex hormone binding globulin SHBG this lowers oestrogen and testosterone thereby increasing osteoporosis risk.

If your body is producing high levels of stress hormones like cortisol then this diminishes testosterone production again increasing risk.

High levels of free radicals (very reactive species with an unpaired electron) are also a contributing factor.

What is the solution?

Like every other disease process there is no singular cause and no singular cure. A multi-faceted approach is needed.

Make sure you are getting adequate vitamins and minerals needed for bone formation. At a minimum get your vitamin D levels, Magnesium and Zinc status checked.

Make sure you are eating enough fats as this is essential to absorb vitamin D and Vitamin K.

Take steps to reduce inflammation (see inflammation section)

Reduce the formation of AGEs (see inflammation section) and make sure your blood sugar is regulated by eating a macronutrient ratio suitable to your metabolic type.

Make sure you are getting a wide range of anti-oxidants in your diet to offset oxidative stress. This can be achieved by eating a wide range of different coloured fruits and vegetables.

Get your hormones tested: testosterone, the various oestrogens and SHBG to assess your risk. Many labs now do Osteoporosis risk assessment profiles. Ask your health care provider about these.

Learn how to weight train correctly and intensely as this type of training is best for increasing bone density.

Pilates training can be very useful to gain better balance and stability essential to reduce risk of falls. I can't count the number of clients who have told me that Pilates training literally saved their asses from potential serious falls due to much improved balance.

Persons with Osteopenia (a precursor to Osteoporosis) and Osteoporosis need to avoid flexion exercises. One study showed an 89% increase in compression fractures during flexion movements[13]. This includes lateral or side bending flexion. Flexion with rotation is also contraindicated. Exercises can be done with a neutral spine.

Extension exercises are also favourable as persons with stronger back extensors have fewer vertebral fractures and better bone density[14,15].

If in doubt pick up a Pilates DVD that's specifically geared towards osteoporosis suffers. Alternatively get one to one training with a fitness professional who has experience with this issue.

With any of my clients who have come to me with existing osteopenia or osteoporosis I have used a combination of Pilates, weight training, nutrition, stress reduction and supplementation. In most cases the bone density went up and at a minimum it did not deteriorate if the client was compliant to the guidelines. Regular bone density scans are essential to keep track of the disease and to see if your interventions are working.

On the energetic level your bones represent that which supports you, standing in your power, standing up for yourself and trusting that the Universe and the process of life itself has your back. Women have traditionally been the nurturers and support givers to others and because of this they may find it difficult to receive support.

This is also affecting men. They too are feeling the stresses and strains of modern living and may also feel unsupported. Also men find it even more difficult to reach out for help if they require it.

The ideal scenario leads one to be able to stand on one's own two feet and at the same time be willing to ask for help when required. It's like the delicate balance of bone building and bone dissolving itself. Too much of one and not enough of the other leads to bone loss. If you try to do everything yourself or you abdicate responsibility and try to get others to do everything for you a lack of equilibrium arises and this lack of equilibrium can show up in your body as bone loss.

Obesity

Obesity is a worldwide epidemic that seems to be growing by the day.

Statistics:

Worldwide obesity has nearly doubled since 1980.

In 2008, more than 1.4 billion adults, 20 and older, were overweight. Of these over 200 million men and nearly 300 million women were obese.

35% of adults aged 20 and over were overweight in 2008, and 11% were obese.

65% of the world's population live in countries where overweight and obesity kills more people than underweight.

More than 40 million children under the age of 5 were overweight or obese in 2012 [16].

The causes of it are extremely complex and individualised including;

Modern diets being highly refined and processed and high calorie

Nutrient deficiency

Sedentary lifestyles

High levels of stress

High levels of toxicity

Emotional eating

Hormonal derangement.

The solution for this problems lies with an individualised approach for each person in question. In over 12 years running my practice these are the elements that I have found work best for my clients:

1. Eat a natural unrefined and unprocessed diet individualised to your metabolic type.

2. Learn the process of biofeedback to fine tune what your body requires and how much it requires. Nutrition is both an art and a science.

3. Get tested as much as possible to help you to individualise your personal healing process. These tests may include comprehensive blood chemistry, hormonal balance, toxicity, allergy and food sensitivity, stool testing for pathogens. These are just a sample of the tests that may be required to unravel your personal obesity generators.

One of my clients had chronic high levels of lead in her body and she could not lose fat till she started to get the lead out. She grew up near a lead mine.

4. Take steps to manage your stress levels. The number one cause of excess weight and obesity I see in my practice is excessively high stress levels. People burning the candle at both ends, all work and no play, too many responsibilities coupled with too much doing and not enough being all generate a recipe for fat storage. As one of my mentors used to say:

> "You're a human being not a human doing"!
> Dr Clifford Oliver

The stress management and supplement sections in this book will be very helpful. Make sure the exercise type you choose is not going to push your stress levels over the edge. Pilates and bioenergetic exercises with stretching for many are the most important starting points. Lifting heavier weights with longer rest intervals is also more favourable. Long steady state aerobics should be avoided by this population.

5: Get counselling or therapy to understand your reasons for overeating and self-sabotage practices.

What drives Obesity on an energetic level?

There are many reasons:

- Attempting to feel more grounded.

- Making yourself a bigger presence in the world so as to feel more substantial and safer.

- Erecting a physical barrier to keep the rest of the world out.

- Some victims of sexual assault realise through therapy that their excess weight was an attempt to desexualise themselves as a form of protection.

- Sometimes the excess weight is a defence against feeling our feelings.

Food is a powerful tool for "numbing out" from the stresses and emotional strains of this reality.

Food can be a rebellion against control. Many people live such structured, programmed and scheduled lives that their only wriggle room for freedom becomes food.

Underweight

Being underweight, while far less common, can have its roots in digestive issues, parasites, over exercising, not doing the right exercise, hormonal and or neurotransmitter imbalance leading to low appetite. Severe food restriction like anorexia or orthorexia (obsessing about food quality and the inherent healthiness or unhealthiness of food) can cause a person to be underweight.

Again being underweight can simply be a form of feeling in control and feeling secure. It can also be a false sense of superiority that masks underlying low self-esteem.

Some people who appear underweight are perfectly healthy. Their genetics have created very small slight bodies. As long as the person feels energised, healthy and happy and their body chemistry and physiology is not suffering there is no need to worry. The worry arises when persons starve themselves to achieve tiny bodies that are not natural for the individual.

Solution:

If you are happy with your body size and healthy you need do nothing. If you are unhappy then I suggest the following:

1. Start a weight training routine which will allow you to put on healthy lean tissue in the form of muscle.

2. Get your digestion assessed with a healthcare practitioner. You may need a stool test or a test to see if you are absorbing food properly.

3. Eliminate foods that sabotage your appetite, sugary snacks and too much coffee as examples.

4. Eat calorie rich nutrient dense foods like nuts, dried fruit, avocado and muscle building protein rich foods.

5. Get a nutritionist to devise a food plan for you calculating your caloric and macronutrient requirements. You may be eating far less than you realise.

6. Eliminate aerobic exercise.

7. Consider hiring a trainer to put you through your weight training sessions. You have to work really out of your comfort zone to build muscle!

8. Consider adding some whey shakes to increase your daily caloric total. You can add carbs to these shakes post workout to replenish your glycogen.

9. Make sure you include starchy carbohydrates which are unrefined in your eating plan. Surges of insulin are required to build muscle. Examples include brown rice, sweet potato, regular potato, and gluten free grains like certified gluten free oats.

10. Manage your stress levels. High levels of stress hormones are very catabolic (tissue wasting). Certain individuals totally lose their appetite when stressed.

High Blood Pressure

Blood pressure is generated by the pumping action of the heart and how readily that blood can flow through the arteries. If the arterial muscles contract or if they are lined with atherosclerosis (plaque) the blood pressure can become higher than normal or desirable. There are differing categories of blood pressure from normal to severely high. High blood pressure is known as hypertension. There are different stages of hypertension with stage one being diagnosed as a diastolic pressure of 90-99 mmHg and a systolic reading of 140-159 mmHg. For a fuller understanding of the range of blood pressure categories please go to: www.heart.org and key in blood pressure.

Stress, lack of exercise, obesity, smoking and excessive alcohol consumption are all known to be contributing factors to high blood pressure. In a seminar with Dr Mark Huston MD, Director of the Hypertension institute of Nashville, some years ago I learned of many other risk factors. These are the main areas Dr Huston addressed:

Excess caffeine consumption (for those who metabolise caffeine slowly from their livers; see section on genetic testing)

Low levels of key nutrients including vitamin C, D, E, Magnesium, Co-Q10, lycopene (a red pigment found in tomatoes).

Elevated levels of iron in the blood

Elevated levels of uric acid

Excessive consumption of trans fats

For a more detailed look at the causes and treatment of hypertension please read Dr Houstons excellent book:

"What your Doctor may not tell you about heart disease"

The above book is an excellent reference for anyone interested in overall heart health and not just blood pressure.

The energetic causes of high blood pressure have to do with mental, emotional or spiritual concerns that impact on a person's physiology. The study of *psychoneuroimmunology* in western medicine is the closest we come to understanding these phenomena.

According to Louise L Hay who has been investigating the mental and emotional patterns behind disease for over 3 decades now hypertension arises from a:

"Longstanding emotional problem that has not been solved"

From the book: "You can heal your life"

What are the solutions to high blood pressure?

According to Dr Mark Huston Hypertension is "a complex disease caused by a constellation of factors"

Therefore a disease that is so complex requires a multi-pronged approach to its resolution.

1. Start a strategy to reduce stress. Many examples are given in this book (chapter 7, Dealing with the fight/flight or freeze response).

2. Consult an exercise professional to devise a weight training program for you. Even though blood pressure goes up during a weight training session overall a person's blood pressure comes down over a period of weeks.

   In one study 15 middle aged men with high blood pressure were put through a weight training routine for the prescribed period. At the end of the 12 weeks both systolic and diastolic readings went down 16 and 12 mmHg respectively[17].

3. Clean up your diet. Try eating for your metabolic type or try the **DASH (dietary approaches to stop hypertension)** nutritional protocol. This is a low sodium plan with emphasis on fruits vegetables and lean proteins.

4. Avoid trans fats from fast food, baked goods and deep fried foods. One web site that gives

information and meal plans for the DASH protocol is www.foods-that-lowerbloodpressure.com

5. Switch from using refined table salt that your purchase at the supermarket to unrefined natural salts like Himalayan or Celtic Sea salt. The salt has a more intense taste so you will use less. It also contains trace minerals which the body requires which are missing in refined table salt.

6. Consider supplementing your diet with some heart healthy nutrients like omega 3 fatty acids found in fish oil, garlic, hawthorn, CoQ10, Resveratrol. Consult your Doctor or health care practitioner for appropriate dosages and to make sure no nutrients you take will contraindicate your medication.

7. Focus on getting more work/life balance. Find time to do things you love.

8. Consider your emotional health. Make time to talk to a therapist, explore your daily feelings by journaling them, do some belly breathing and see what feelings arise. Then watch those feelings leave.

9. If you are taking a multivitamin make sure it is iron free.

10. Are you a type A personality or a perfectionist or someone who always needs to be in control? I have seen this with many hypertensive clients. Learn how to delegate and learn how to switch off at the end of the day.

Chapter 13

Final thoughts

Emotional Density of the Root Chakra

The root chakra is described as being the most energetically dense of all the chakras. This energetic density manifests itself as matter; the muscles, bones, cells and fluids of the human body. This energetic density also manifests itself as very intense emotions. The emotions of the root chakra are some of the most difficult of the human condition:

Fear, Rage, Fury , Hate, Guilt, Humiliation, Blame, Shame, Regret, Feeling Abandoned , Apathy, Loneliness , Emptiness and Devastation are all some of the really heavy and challenging emotions of this chakra.

Can we love our selves through all of these emotions? Every emotion that is avoided is like a little child who has been abandoned and is longing to come home, be loved and accepted. Many addictions and dysfunctional behaviours of the root chakra stem from unwillingness to acknowledge, fully feel and love those parts of ourselves that have felt this way at one time or another on our journey. If we can fully feel these feelings as they arise in our lives then they can be transformed and returned to love. Fear is Love in disguise. Hate is love in disguise.

Once you transform these emotions you come out the other side with a sense of Peace, Serenity, Security, Surrender and a Trust that life and the process of living ultimately has your back.

This is the theory at any rate! In practice the drama and trauma of the root chakra represents some of the most debilitating, gut wrenching and devastating aspects of the human condition. I was listening to a radio show one day and a caller was looking for some insight into his obesity. His entire family, wife and two kids, had been killed in a car crash some years earlier.

Where this guy was finding the will to live astounded the hosts of the show and I dare say a fair few listeners as well. How can you choose to live on after such devastation? Many do not and suicide is their choice.

On another occasion I visited an art gallery and was mesmerised by the beautiful works on display which were all landscapes with an interpretation of light. It reminded me of the work of 18th century artist William Turner. I got talking to the artist and I found out his son had committed suicide some years earlier. His devastation was apparent, however more serenity came through than anything else. He said he painted his way through the tragedy. Every person who walked into his gallery was being changed and uplifted by his paintings. They were other worldly and transformative.

If you have the courage and somewhere find the fortitude to move through the devastation then you arrive at serenity. You start to live your life not from a place of avoidance but from a place of trust that whatever happens you can cope, survive and move through it.

"Joy and woe are woven fine,
A clothing for the soul divine.
Under every grief and pine
Runs a joy with silken twine."

From Auguries of Innocence, a poem by William Blake

So if you have experienced great loss, or are feeling suicidal or you have been diagnosed with a life threatening disease or you are lost in pain and disease just remember you are at the bottom of the barrel of the human condition. If you can find a way to hang on and move through it perhaps you may find the joy that is woven through your sorrow.

Environmental Consciousness

With the root chakra comes our connection to Mother Earth. This can come in the form of a love of nature or animals. It can come in the form of environmental activism on a small or large scale. You could join Green peace or simply decide to recycle as much of your waste as possible. You may decide to use biodegradable washing powder. You could start to use eco conscious cosmetics. Maybe you will decide to make sure that your food is as locally sourced as possible and organic.

All of these behaviours are showing an evolving consciousness that we are one with the earth. If the Body represents the microcosm then the Earth represents the macrocosm. People who eat low quality, processed and toxic foods will be very unlikely to be environmentally conscious. People who nourish their bodies with high quality vitality giving foods are more likely to care for the earth. It's not a co-incidence that the earth is plagued by masses of pollution and at the same time we are experiencing a global crisis of obesity. The outer toxicity is mirroring the inner pollution.

To boost your root chakra consider becoming more environmentally aware. At the very minimum using ecological products will cut down on your overall body burden of toxins and this is very good news for the body. Many persons have excess weight or suffer from obesity simply because they are riddled with toxins. In an ideal world the body eliminates toxins itself easily however these toxins are overwhelming in the modern era and they create poorly and overloaded organs of elimination. The first rule of thumb is to reduce the input of toxins into the system.

Parasympathetic versus Sympathetic Nervous System

The body's nervous system is extremely complicated. In a nutshell it's divided into two main wings; the central nervous system, **CNS** (brain and spinal cord) and the peripheral nervous system, **PNS,** (which are all of the nerves arising from the spinal cord). The peripheral nervous system is itself comprised of two wings. One of those wings is called the Autonomic Nervous System, **ANS.**

The autonomic nervous system controls all of those things which happen subconsciously. So the autonomic system is like an automatic system that gets vital functions done without thinking. It too is divided into two main wings; the Parasympathetic system and the Sympathetic system.

The Parasympathetic system is responsible for what is often called the "rest and digest" functions and the Sympathetic side is often referred to as the "Fight or Flight" system.

In simplified terms the sympathetic nervous system gets you up, mobilised and going and it really ramps things up if there is an emergency. It does things like dilate your pupils so you can see better, and it inhibits peristalsis (the natural muscular contractions along the gut wall). Who has time to poop when you are running from a sabre toothed tiger? It increases your heart rate, it gets your lungs absorbing more oxygen and it increases sweating so you can stay cool when you're on the run. Basically it's a system of go, go, go!

The parasympathetic nervous system on the other hand is designed to bring you back to balance after all the get up and go of the sympathetic side of things. It is responsible for digestion and defecation and aspects of sexual arousal.

The sympathetic nervous system is tissue wasting (catabolic). It is responsible for the feeling of an adrenaline rush. The parasympathetic nervous system is tissue building (anabolic) and it is responsible for repairing and healing the body. Both sides of the system complement each other. When one side is working the other is not. You cannot be in a fight or flight mode and a rest and digest mode at the same time. The problem with modern living is that many individuals spend most of their time in sympathetic mode. It's go, go, go, action and doing all the time. Then the same person trains for a marathon to "relax" and switch off. This individuals mind may be switched on to something else however their body is still in a state of sympathetic dominance! In time this leads to burn out, adrenal fatigue and thyroid disorders among other issues.

How do you know if you are stressed? Sympathetic Dominance.

In my experience working with clients one to one for 12+ years most individuals who are highly stressed don't even realise they are stressed. They usually come to me for a number of reasons. The most obvious ones being:

1. An inability to lose fat or "weight", especially around the belly area, regardless of eating well and exercising.
2. Complaining of fatigue.

3. Joint pain with back ache being the most common.

What these individuals have not realised is that they have been in flight or fight mode for years and in many cases decades.

What are the other signs of sympathetic dominance?

4. Dilated pupils resulting in sensitivity to bright light.
5. Ongoing worry or anxiety.
6. Possible panic attacks.
7. Inability to relax and unwind.
8. Disturbed sleep.
9. Indigestion.
10. Constipation.
11. Depression. High cortisol levels (a stress hormone) wipe out serotonin the neurotransmitter of happiness.
12. Weakened immune system. You catch every bug going.
13. Low sex drive.
14. Stomach ulcers.
15. Cravings for sweets/alcohol/cigarettes or coffee. These are all potent modulators of blood sugar. Blood sugar regulation is knocked off kilter with chronic stress.
16. Chronic muscle tension.

17. Water retention or Oedema.
18. Being on the go constantly. Not being able to simply do nothing.
19. Feeling guilty if you are not busy all the time.
20. Sinus problems eg post nasal drip.
21. Early morning waking (waking before 5 am).
22. Bilateral weakness of the adductor or inner thigh muscles.
23. Persistent or nagging injuries that just don't seem to respond to treatment.

What do you do if you realise you are sympathetic dominant?

1. Start eating an unrefined, unprocessed, organic diet ideally individualised for your metabolic type.

2. Many individuals with sympathetic dominance have blood sugar disturbances so small frequent meals may be best for you.

3. Try the stress reduction techniques in chapter 7. You need to do something daily.

4. Reconsider your working environment. Do you need to delegate more? Stand up to the workplace bully? Leave work at the office? Ask for more support or change jobs completely? The important thing is not to make any rash decisions. One way of finding a job you would love is to read the book:

"Finding Your Element: How to Discover Your Talents and Passions and Transform Your Life" by Ken Robinson

5. Start a hobby.

6. Try some of the supplements for the root chakra.

7. Get an adrenal stress profile tested by a laboratory. You will need a health care practitioner to order and interpret the test for you. It will let you know what stage you are at regards stress and some tests give additional information. You can then begin a program of customised nutrition and supplementation.

8. Make more time for friends and family and social life in general.

9. Schedule regular holidays and be sure to take them. Do not bring work on holidays.

10. Get counselling or therapy for any unresolved emotional issues.

11. Dance.

12. Try art therapy, writing poetry or some craft. This will get you out of your mathematical logical brain and into the artistic creative brain. For many this is enough to restore balance.

13. Establish a regular sleep routine getting to bed by 10 pm if possible.

14. Schedule regular massage or some type of body therapy to support relaxation e.g. sauna therapy or Hydrotherapy.

15. Anytime you feel stressed slow down your breathing. It can change your energy and outlook in an instant.

Other techniques to restore the root chakra

1. Stay in tune with the circadian rhythm. This is the natural cycle of night and day that is accompanied by a specific pattern in the secretion of cortisol. This is largely what is tested in an adrenal stress index. Your cortisol should rise slowly at about 6am and reach a peek around 12pm. It should then slowly decline from 12pm onwards allowing the body to wind down and naturally prepare for sleep. Try to stay in tune with this rhythm and try not to get up earlier than 6am or go to bed later than 10pm. This may be slightly adjusted depending on what part of the world you live in. When I go on holidays to Arizona I end up going to bed really early as sunset is around 8pm. I do however get up earlier as sun rise is around 5am. Try to get up at the same time every day and go to bed at the same time. This supports the body's natural rhythm and is in keeping with the earth's rhythm.

2. Try aromatherapy in various forms from massage to hot baths with added oils to using a diffuser with the oils in your home. Sent is the sense of the root chakra. Any oil extracted from trees is excellent for grounding. The trees roots go deep into the earth. One of my favourites is sandalwood. It is used in Ayurveda for stress and anxiety. Vetiver, Ylang- Ylang, Cedar wood and Patchouli are also excellent grounders. Rose oil has been shown to be a great stress fighter.

"Fragrance inhalation of rose oil or patchouli oil caused a 40% decrease in relative sympathetic activity......

while fragrance inhalation of rose oil caused a 30% decrease in adrenaline concentration[1]."

One of the ways to use the oils is to put them in a spray bottle (added to water) and simply mist your energy field with them.

In another study on Ylang-Ylang

"The present results demonstrated that inhalation of Ylang-Ylang Aroma (YYA) significantly decreased the systolic and diastolic blood pressure. The present results show a sedative effect of YYA and this study provides some evidences for the usage of YYA in medicinal agent[2].

3. Colour therapy can be used to support the root chakra. The colour of the root chakra is red. You can use this to your advantage by wearing red clothing to give you an energy boost or maybe the edge in performance! Sounds strange? A 2005 study has shown a statistical difference in sports performance with athletes wearing red attire winning more frequently.

"Red coloration is a sexually selected, testosterone-dependent signal of male quality in a variety of animals, and in some non-human species a male's dominance can be experimentally increased by attaching artificial red stimuli......... a similar effect can influence the outcome of physical contests in humans — across a range of sports, we find that wearing red is consistently associated with a higher probability of winning[3]."

The root chakra is the chakra of power, strength, physicality and sex drive and testosterone is one of the principal hormones connected to it. Maybe that's why women wear red lipstick or a red dress is perceived as having more sexual allure. Red after all is the colour of passion.

If a person is filled with rage, an excess energy of the base chakra, red would not be a great colour. It would be like a red flag before a bull.

Red light therapy is becoming very popular in the beauty industry to heal skin, reduce wrinkles and treat acne. This red light is from the visible spectrum of light as opposed to the infrared light which is invisible.

Your Money Flow and the Root Chakra

Our root chakra is the chakra of survival and in this day and age we need money to survive. It puts a roof over our heads and food on the table, all reptilian needs. So if your financial flow is not what you would like it to be in spite of "doing the leg work" then you need to look at what might be blocking your root chakra.

The number 1 thing that blocks people's money flow is beliefs around money. "Money is the root of all evil" and "Filthy Rich" are examples of expressions that convey our mistrust about money and the fact that many of us suspect that it's not very spiritual to have or pursue money.

These of course are just beliefs. Money, like everything else, is just energy. And energy is not good or bad or evil for that matter! Money in many ways represents the flow of energy into your life.

Our beliefs around money largely come from our parents. If your parents had a poverty consciousness or believed in lack and struggle or believed that money was the root of all evil then don't be surprised if you struggle with money. Look at all of the beliefs around money that you inherited from your parents and then erase them.

What beliefs did you pick up from society? List all of those and erase them too. Many people have gotten killed for money, they attract more attention when they have money, people try to swindle you when you have money, and in-laws fight over inheritances. All of these scenarios can make people believe that money is bad news and that you're better off with just enough to survive. Review those beliefs. Are they working for you? If not erase them from your mind.

If you don't look after your physical body then don't be surprised if your money flow is not amazing or at the very least you have no ease around money. What I mean regarding ease around money is that you need to be able to enjoy it. Enjoy the gifts and ease and comfort and opportunities it brings into your life.

I have had many clients over the years that were very wealthy and still struggled with money. They either never had enough, they over worked to get money to the detriment of their health, or they were always fearful they would lose it. All these individuals had weak or blocked root chakras. In contrast I have had clients over a period of years and as their root chakras developed (through great nutrition, exercise, stress relief and exercises from this book) I could sense their ease around money improving. They started to pay me on time and didn't complain about my fees! Great news all round! Persons with weak root chakras are always penny pinching. They will always want something for nothing.

I remember many years ago a guy called Bill Phillips started what was to become a world-wide phenomenon; The Physique Transformation contest. He got thousands of individuals from all over the United States to eat a bodybuilding style diet and lift weights and add some cardio over a 12 week period. He also got these people to write essays about their transformations. I loved reading the transformations as you got to see the trials and tribulations and successes of these people.

One of the most outstanding constants in the transformation stories was an increase in money flow for many contestants. The women got leaner and usually smaller and the men got leaner and more muscular. Research shows that slender women get paid more and also more well-built guys earn more and that for both sexes obesity (a dysfunction of the root chakra) caused both sexes to earn less money[4].

If your motivation to get up and go and take action is low then consider giving your dopamine a boost. Reread the section:

Dopamine; the neurotransmitter of Motivation and Drive! From chapter 10 on mindfulness about your behavior.

Your Home and the health of your Root Chakra

Since the root chakra is concerned with safety and security, your home, and how you keep it, has a great influence on the health of this chakra. The ancient science of Fung Shui is a classic example of how adjusting your environment can affect everything from health to money flow and abundance.

"I don't have to believe in Feng Shui, but I use it because it makes me money."

Donald Trump

If your home is filled with clutter, you are in an energetic mess that drains your energy. Try a bit of spring cleaning and get rid of things you do not use on a regular basis.
Keep worktops clear. Make sure each room gets enough light and ventilation.
Make sure your home is aesthetically pleasing to you. This covers the nurturing aspects of the root chakra. Your outer environment is a mirror of your interiority. So if you wish to create a shift on the inside, working on your home can be a powerful tool.

Geopathic Stress
Geopathic stress is the study of the earth energies and their effect on our wellbeing. The earth emits natural electromagnetic radiation. Geopathic stress is a distortion of this natural radiation as a result of underground water currents, mineral deposits, geological fault lines and lines of energy known as Hartmann lines (Named after the German Doctor , Earnest Hartmann, MD, who discovered them) .
Feng shui masters from the east have known for millennia the importance of these energy currents and how to work with them or avoid them for health , wealth and harmony.
"Certain locations (stress zones; geopathy) affect human beings and animals. Such places can induce stress, hamper sleep quality and quality of life, can lead to decreased melatonin concentrations, diminish our resistance on infections, appear to

influence aging and work performance in the long term."[5]

So what can you do about geopathic stress? The research in western science is in the early days as instruments are being developed to test it and modify it. From the eastern traditions, Shamen, Feng Shui practitioners and dowsers may be able to help you. I had my home cleared by a space clearing specialist and most definitely felt and perceived the benefits pretty much instantly.

For more reading on geopathic stress see:

"Geopathic Stress Zones and Their Influence on the Human Organism"[6]

Electromagnetic Fields

We are all swimming in a sea of electromagnetic fields on a daily basis. TVs, lighting, mobile phones, tablets, and other electronic gadgets all are emitting electrical and magnetic fields that can disturb your body's energy field. This can lead to sleep disturbance, immunosuppression, abnormal gene transcription, reduction in free radical scavengers (particularly melatonin), neurotoxicity in humans and animals, carcinogenicity in humans, serious impacts on human and animal sperm morphology and function and effects on brain and cranial bone development in the offspring of animals that are exposed to cell phone radiation during pregnancy[7].

Ways to Reduce Electromagnetic Radiation

1. Unplug all electrical devices in your bedroom at night or switch them off at the plug socket. Remember that even if the light switch is in an off

position your electric device is emitting radiation if it is plugged in.

2. Keep electric devices at least 8 feet from your bed.
3. Use a wind up alarm clock.
4. Do not keep your mobile phone in your bedroom.
5. When using your phone use the speaker phone function or specialized head set for emf reduction.
6. Limit your time using Wi-Fi devices and do not sleep with them in your bedroom.
7. Consider using a grounding cord for your computer to dissipate the emf.
8. Consider using a personal emf protection device like the Q-Link.

Overall guidelines:

In order to get the best out of this book go back to chapter one and the questionnaire to assess your root chakra.

There are 5 sections:

A: Physical Appearance

B: Health

C: Financial Security

D: Family

E: Environmental Consciousness

Identify the area which you wish to start on. If working on your financial security seems too overwhelming then maybe you could start with exercise. If you have a pancake butt maybe you can start with the glute/buttock exercises in this book. If your energy levels are low then maybe you need to tune in to chapter 12 and the fatigue section.

Gradually work your way through all topics in the book. Working on our interpersonal relationships is always one of the toughest things to do as it brings up all of our vulnerabilities and self-judgements. The most important relationship to work on is your relationship with yourself. So if you have not been developing and supporting your own Self Respect, the foundation stone for all healthy relationships, then drop by to chapters 10 and 11 to see if some new awareness can be stimulated. Maybe this could be a call to get some counselling to really address some issues or behaviours that you have been avoiding.

The Root Chakra can be supported from the most basic levels of awareness (eat right for your unique body requirements) to the more advanced (make peace with and heal your core issues: e.g. my relationship with my Mother, my overwhelming need to be a people pleaser).

Healing it is an ongoing process. Your body and your being are never static. You are learning every day; you are expanding in awareness every day. If you make strides to support your root chakra daily your whole life will eventually change. You will find yourself more present, more tolerant and supportive of yourself, more capable and independent, more energised.

You are no longer a victim of the past or anxious about the future because you become physically and energetically capable of living in the present. You are finally living in your own body. Once you are fully anchored in your own body your Feeling, Knowing, Being and Perceiving faculties take over and the Mind becomes the servant of the Spirit working in harmony with the Body. Until then you will always be a slave to your Mind. Your efforts at Mindfulness, Affirmations, the Law of Attraction and the Power of Intention will start to pay off. None of these methods work unless you are actually in your body! Until your root chakra is healed you are not actually in your body.

Being in your body gives you the path towards the greatest empowerment. Working towards healing your Root Chakra is the most effective way of achieving this. Being in your Body means you are fully in alignment and the marriage of Heart and Mind can happen. You develop the capacity to turn your dreams into a reality and your ability to manifest the things you desire in your life happens more quickly.

When you are in your body you have access to the power of NOW. When you are in your body you are PRESENT. When you are in your body you are AWARE (mindful).

The last several hundred years especially since the industrial revolution and the explosion of technology have created a society ruled by the mind and disconnected from the body. The future will be a Body-Centric revolution whereby the wisdom and consciousness that the body facilitates for us will be lauded, esteemed and followed instead of derided, pushed aside and numbed out through alcohol, drugs, over/under eating and over/under exercising.

Being in your body brings a sense of peace, serenity, safety, security, vibrant health, energy , vitality, ability to manifest your dreams, abundance, a foundation for better relationships and a beautiful and healthy body. Are you ready to claim Your Root Power? The choice as always is up to YOU!

References

Chapter 2

1. "Higher antioxidant and lower cadmium concentrations and lower incidence of pesticide residues in organically grown crops: a systematic literature review and meta-analyses". British Journal of Nutrition/ Volume 112 / Issue 05 / September 2014, pp 794-811

2. Rose G, Tunstall-Pedoe HD, Heller RF. UK heart disease prevention project: incidence and mortality results. Lancet 1983;1(8333):1062--6.

3. Kaul N et al, "A comparison of fish oil, flaxseed oil and hempseed oil supplementation on selected parameters of cardiovascular health in healthy volunteers." J AM Coll Nutr, 2008 Feb;27(1):51-8.

4. Das, U. N. (2006), Essential fatty acids: biochemistry, physiology and pathology. Biotechnology Journal, 1: 420–439. doi: 10.1002/biot.200600012

5. Uffe Ravnskov PhD, MD "VARIANCE AND DISSENT A hypothesis out-of-date: The diet–heart idea", Journal of Clinical Epidemiology 55 (2002) 1057–1063

6. Hämäläinen EK et al, "Decrease of serum total and free testosterone during a low-fat high-fibre die"t, Journal of Steroid Biochemistry 1983 Mar;18(3):369-70.

7. Ranieri M et al, The use of alpha-lipoic acid (ALA), gamma linoleic acid (GLA) and rehabilitation in the treatment of back pain: effect on health-related quality of life. *International Journal of Immunopathology and Pharmacology*. 2009. 22(3 Suppl), 45-50.)

8. Whigham et al, Efficacy of conjugated linoleic acid for reducing fat mass: a meta-analysis in humans, *Am J Clin Nutr* May 2007 vol. 85 no. 5 1203-1211

Chapter 3

1. Forbes-Ewan, Chris. Effect of Vegetarian Diets on Performance in Strength Sports. Sport science. 2002, V6.

2. http://www.deakin.edu.au/research/stories/2012/03/20/women-should-eat-red-meat

3. Sleigh, AE, Kuehl KS, Elliot DL. Efficacy of tart cherry juice to reduce inflammation among patients with osteoarthritis. *American College of Sports Medicine Annual Meeting.* May 30, 2012.

4. E.M. Seymour et al, Regular Tart Cherry Intake Alters Abdominal Adiposity, Adipose Gene Transcription, and Inflammation in Obesity-Prone Rats Fed a High Fat Diet, Journal of Medicinal Food. October 2009, 12(5): 935-942. doi:10.1089/jmf.2008.0270.

5. Takanori Tsuda et al, Anthocyanin enhances adipocytokine secretion and adipocyte-specific gene expression in isolated rat adipocytes, Biochem Biophys Res Commun 2004 Mar;316(1):149-57

6. T. Yamauchi et al, The fat-derived hormone adiponectin reverses insulin resistance associated with both lipoatrophy and obesity, Nature Medicine 7, 941 - 946 (2001) doi:10.1038/90984

7. Kikuko Hotta et al, Circulating Concentrations of the Adipocyte Protein Adiponectin Are Decreased in Parallel With Reduced Insulin Sensitivity During the Progression to Type 2 Diabetes in Rhesus Monkeys,

10.2337/diabetes.50.5.1126 *Diabetes May 2001 vol. 50 no. 5* 1126-1133

8. Mari Kannan M et al, Pharmacodynamics of ellagic acid on cardiac troponin-T, lyosomal enzymes and membrane bound ATPases: mechanistic clues from biochemical, cytokine and in vitro studies, Chem Biol Interact. 2011 Sep 5;193(2):154-61. doi: 10.1016/j.cbi.2011.06.005. Epub 2011 Jul 5.

9. Hui Zhang et al, Antitumor effect and mechanism of an ellagic acid derivative on the HepG2 human hepatocellular carcinoma cell line, Oncology Letters, February 2014
Volume 7 Issue 2 ,Print ISSN: 1792-1074

10. Barch DH et al, Ellagic acid induces NAD(P)H:quinone reductase through activation of the antioxidant responsive element of the rat NAD(P)H:quinone reductase gene, Carcinogenesis. 1994 Sep;15(9):2065-8.

11. Umesalma S et al, Differential inhibitory effects of the polyphenol ellagic acid on inflammatory mediators NF-kappaB, iNOS, COX-2, TNF-alpha, and IL-6 in 1,2-dimethylhydrazine-induced rat colon carcinogenesis, Basic Clin Pharmacol Toxicol. 2010 Aug;107(2):650-5. doi: 10.1111/j.1742-7843.2010.00565.x. Epub 2010 Apr 14.

12. Panchal SK, Ward L, Brown L. Ellagic acid attenuates high-carbohydrate, high-fat diet-induced metabolic syndrome in rats. *Eur J Nutr.* Epub 2012 Apr 27

13. Woo A[1], Min B, Ryoo S. Piceatannol-3'-O-beta-D-glucopyranoside as an active component of rhubarb activates endothelial nitric oxide synthase through inhibition of arginase activity. Exp Mol Med. 2010 Jul 31;42(7):524-32.

14. Mohammad Athar et al, Resveratrol: A Review of Pre-clinical Studies for Human Cancer Prevention, Toxicol Appl Pharmacol. Nov 1, 2007; 224(3): 274–283.

15. Samarjit Das et al, Experimental evidence for the cardioprotective effects of red wine, Exp Clin Cardiol. 2007 Spring; 12(1): 5–10.

16. Francesca De Amicis et al, Resveratrol, through NF-Y/p53/Sin3/HDAC1 complex phosphorylation, inhibits estrogen receptor a gene expression via p38^{MAPK}/CK2 signaling in human breast cancer cells, *October 2011 The FASEB Journal vol. 25 no. 10 3695-3707*

17. Lavigne JP et al, [Cranberry (Vaccinium macrocarpon) and urinary tract infections: study model and review of literature], Pathol Biol (Paris). 2007 Nov;55(8-9):460-4. Epub 2007 Oct 1

18. Bonifait L[1], Grenier D., Cranberry polyphenols: potential benefits for dental caries and periodontal disease, J Can Dent Assoc. 2010;76:a130.

19. Yi-Fang Chua, Rui Hai Liua,b,, Cranberries inhibit LDL oxidation and induce LDL receptor expression in hepatocytes, Department of Food Science, Stocking Hall, Cornell University, Ithaca, NY 14853-7201, United States

Institute of Comparative and Environmental Toxicology, Stocking Hall, Cornell University, Ithaca, NY 14853-7201, United States. www.sciencedirect.com

20. Luo Q et al, Lycium barbarum polysaccharides induce apoptosis in human prostate cancer cells and inhibits prostate cancer growth in a xenograft mouse model of human prostate cancer, J Med Food. 2009 Aug;12(4):695-703. doi: 10.1089/jmf.2008.1232.

21. Shan X[1], Zhou J, Ma T, Chai Q., Lycium barbarum polysaccharides reduce exercise-induced oxidative

stress, Int J Mol Sci. 2011 Feb 9;12(2):1081-8. doi: 10.3390/ijms12021081.

22. P.J.D. Bouic et al, The effects of b-sitosterol (BSS) and b-sitosterol glucoside (BSSG) mixture on selected immune parameters of marathon runners: inhibition of post marathon immune suppression and inflammation, International Journal of Sports Medicine, 20: 258-262. 1999.

23. Mahyar Ethminan et al , "The Role of Tomato Products and Lycopene in the Prevention of Prostate Cancer: A Meta-Analysis of Observational Studies", *Cancer Epidemiol Biomarkers Prev March 2004 13;* 340

24. Lu QY et al, Inverse associations between plasma lycopene and other carotenoids and prostate cancer, Cancer Epidemiol Biomarkers Prev. 2001 Jul;10(7):749-56.

25. Giovannucci E et al, A prospective study of tomato products, lycopene, and prostate cancer risk, J Natl Cancer Inst. 2002 Mar 6;94(5):391-8.

26. Dewanto V et al, Thermal processing enhances the nutritional value of tomatoes by increasing total antioxidant activity, J Agric Food Chem. 2002 May 8;50(10):3010-4.

27. Mats Harms-Ringdahl et al, Tomato juice intake suppressed serum concentration of 8-oxodG after extensive physical activity, Nutrition Journal 2012, 11:29 doi:10.1186/1475-2891-11-29

Chapter 4

1. Joy L Frestedt et al, A whey-protein supplement increases fat loss and spares lean muscle in obese subjects: a randomized human clinical study, Nutr Metab (Lond). 2008; 5: 8.

2. Padayatty SJ et al, Human adrenal glands secrete vitamin C in response to adrenocorticotrophic hormone, Am J Clin Nutr. 2007 Jul;86(1):145-9.

3. Huck et al, Vitamin C status and perception of effort during exercise in obese adults adhering to a calorie-reduced diet, nutritionjournal.com, January 2012

4. Arakawa M et al, The effects of branched-chain amino acid granules on the accumulation of tissue triglycerides and uncoupling proteins in diet-induced obese mice, Endocr J. 2011;58(3):161-70. Epub 2011 Mar 1.

5. Qin LQ et al, Higher branched-chain amino acid intake is associated with a lower prevalence of being overweight or obese in middle-aged East Asian and Western adults, J Nutr. 2011 Feb;141(2):249-54. doi: 10.3945/jn.110.128520. Epub 2010 Dec 15.

6. Yiying Zhang et al, Increasing Dietary Leucine Intake Reduces Diet-Induced Obesity and Improves Glucose and Cholesterol Metabolism in Mice via Multimechanisms, *Diabetes June 2007 vol. 56 no. 6 1647-1654*

7. Sharp CP, Pearson DR, Amino acid supplements and recovery from high-intensity resistance training, J Strength Cond Res. 2010 Apr;24(4):1125-30.

8. Alessandra Valerio, Giuseppe D'Antona, and Enzo Nisoli, Branched-chain amino acids, mitochondrial biogenesis, and healthspan: an evolutionary perspective, Aging (Albany NY). May 2011; 3(5): 464–478.

9. Ralph J. Manders et al, Insulinotropic and Muscle Protein Synthetic Effects of Branched-Chain Amino Acids: Potential Therapy for Type 2 Diabetes and Sarcopenia, Nutrients. Nov 2012; 4(11): 1664–1678.

10. Ram Chandra Saxena et al, Efficacy of an Extract of *Ocimum tenuiflorum* (OciBest) in the Management of General Stress: A Double-Blind, Placebo-Controlled Study, Evid Based Complement Alternat Med. 2012; 2012: 894509.

11. Priyabrata Pattanayak et al, *Ocimum sanctum* Linn. A reservoir plant for therapeutic applications: An overview, Pharmacogn Rev. 2010 Jan-Jun; 4(7): 95–105.

12. Raut AA et al, Exploratory study to evaluate tolerability, safety, and activity of Ashwagandha (Withania somnifera) in healthy volunteers, J Ayurveda Integr Med. 2012 Jul;3(3):111-4.

13. Van Wietmarschen HA et al, Evaluation of symptom, clinical chemistry and metabolomics profiles during Rehmannia six formula (R6) treatment: an integrated and personalized data analysis approach, J Ethnopharmacol. 2013 Dec 12;150(3):851-9.

14. Vazeille E et al, Curcumin treatment prevents increased proteasome and apoptosome activities in rat skeletal muscle during reloading and improves subsequent recovery, J Nutr Biochem. 2012 Mar;23(3):245-51

15. Kim T et al, Curcumin activates AMPK and suppresses gluconeogenic gene expression in hepatoma cells, Biochem Biophys Res Commun. 2009 Oct 16;388(2):377-82

16. Asma Ejaz et al, Curcumin Inhibits Adipogenesis in 3T3-L1 Adipocytes and Angiogenesis and Obesity in C57/BL Mice J. Nutr. May 2009 139: 919-925.

17. Binu Chandran, and Ajay Goel, A Randomized, Pilot Study to Assess the Efficacy and Safety of Curcumin in

Patients with Active Rheumatoid Arthritis, Phytother. Res. (2012)

18. Belcaro et al, Efficacy and safety of Meriva®, a curcumin-phosphatidylcholine complex, during extended administration in osteoarthritis patients, Altern Med Rev. 2010 Dec;15(4):337-44.

19. Guo H et al, Curcumin induces cell cycle arrest and apoptosis of prostate cancer cells by regulating the expression of IkappaBalpha, c-Jun and androgen receptor, Pharmazie. 2013 Jun;68(6):431-4.

20. Olsson EM et al, A randomised, double-blind, placebo-controlled, parallel-group study of the standardised extract shr-5 of the roots of Rhodiola rosea in the treatment of subjects with stress-related fatigue, Planta Med. 2009 Feb;75(2):105-12

21. Van Diermen D et al, Monoamine oxidase inhibition by Rhodiola rosea L. roots, J Ethnopharmacol. 2009 Mar 18;122(2):397-401

Chapter 7

1. Heitmann BL, Frederiksen P, "Thigh circumference and risk of heart disease and premature death: prospective cohort study." BMJ. 2009 Sep 3;339:b3292. doi: 10.1136/bmj.b3292.

2. Miho Nagasawa et al, "Dog's gaze at its owner increases owner's urinary oxytocin during social interaction", Hormones and Behavior 55 (2009) 434–441

3. Heinrichs M et al, "Social support and oxytocin interact to suppress cortisol and subjective responses to psychosocial stress." Biol Psychiatry. 2003 Dec 15;54(12):1389-98.

4. Gaétan Chevalier et al, " Earthing (Grounding) the Human Body Reduces BloodViscosity—a Major

Factor in Cardiovascular Disease", The Journal of alternative and complementary medicine volume 19, number 2, 2013, pp. 102–110.

5. Karol Sokal et al , " Earthing the Human Body Influences Physiologic Processes", The Journal of alternative and complementary medicine, volume 17, number 4, 2011, pp. 301–308

Chapter 9

1. Katherine Harmon, " The Mother –Baby bond", Scientific American .com , May 6th , 2010

2. Weaver et al, "Epigenetic programming by maternal behaviour", Nature Neuroscience 7, 847 - 854 (2004)

3. Cornelis et al, Coffee, CYP1A2 genotype, and risk of myocardial infarction, JAMA. 2006 Mar 8;295(10):1135-41.

4. From Quantum Physics: What is Real, Scientific American, August 2013

5. From the Book by Carl Jung: The development of personality

6. Book of Exodus 20:5

7. From "The merchant of Venice".

8. Blog post "Unlived lives" from www.awakeninthedream.com

9. From the book: Visions

Chapter 10

1. *Source: psychologytoday.com*

2. Georgiadis JR and Holstege G. "Human brain activation during sexual stimulation of the penis." J Comp Neurol. 2005 Dec 5;493(1):33-8.

3. Source: Psychology Today

Chapter 11

1. Source: the free dictionary

Chapter 12

1. Vallfors B. Acute, "Subacute and Chronic Low Back Pain: Clinical Symptoms, Absenteeism and Working Environment." Scan J Rehab Med Suppl 1985; 11: 1-98.

2. http://growingstronger.nutrition.tufts.edu/why_grow_stronger/benefits.html

3. Unal et al, "The role of clinical pilates exercises in children with juvenile idiopathic arthritis: a pilot study", Pediatr Rheumatol Online J. 2011; 9(Suppl 1): P117.

4. Neilan et al, "Myocardial injury and ventricular dysfunction related to training levels among nonelite participants in the Boston marathon." Circulation,2006 Nov 28;114(22):2325-33. Epub 2006 Nov 13.

5. Siegel et al, "Effect of marathon running on inflammatory and hemostatic markers.", The American Journal of Cardiology[2001, 88(8):918-20, A9]

6. Slavicha GM, et al "Neural sensitivity to social rejection is associated with infammatory responses to social stress" *Proc Natl Acad Sci* 2010; DOI: 10.1073/pnas.1009164107.

7. MARTHA K. MCCLINTOCK, "Menstrual Synchrony and Suppression", *Nature* 229, 244 - 245 (22 January 1971); doi:10.1038/229244a0

8. Pimentel M et al, "Eradication of small intestinal bacterial overgrowth reduces symptoms of irritable bowel syndrome", Am J Gastroenterol. 2000 Dec;95(12):3503-6.

9. Ringel-Kulka et al, "The clinical effectiveness of probiotics in irritable bowel syndrome." J Clin Gastroenterology. 2011 Nov;45 Suppl:S145-8. doi: 10.1097/MCG.0b013e31822d32d3.

10. Ringel-Kulka et al, "Probiotic bacteria Lactobacillus acidophilus NCFM and Bifidobacterium lactis Bi-07 versus placebo for the symptoms of bloating in patients with functional bowel disorders: a double-blind study", J Clin Gastroenterol. 2011 Jul;45(6):518-25. doi: 10.1097/MCG.0b013e31820ca4d6.

11. Culligan PJ et al, "A randomized clinical trial comparing pelvic floor muscle training to a Pilates exercise program for improving pelvic muscle strength", Int Urogynecol J. 2010 Apr;21(4):401-8. doi: 10.1007/s00192-009-1046-z. Epub 2010 Jan 22.

12. Source: Harvard School of public Health.

13. Sinaki, M., & Mikkelsen, B.A. "Postmenopausal spinal osteoporosis: Flexion versus extension exercises", Arch Phys Med Rehabil. 1984 Oct;65(10):593-6.

14. Sinaki et al, "Can strong back extensors prevent vertebral fractures in women with osteoporosis?", Mayo Clin Proc. 1996 Oct;71(10):951-6.

15. Sinaki, M, et al. " Stronger back muscles reduce the incidence of vertebral fractures: A prospective 10 year follow-up of postmenopausal women". Bone, 2002, Jun;30(6):836-41.

16. Source: World Health Organisation   www.who.int

17. Moraes et al, "Effect of 12 weeks of resistance exercise on post-exercise hypotension in stage 1 hypertensive individuals" , J Hum Hypertens. 2012 Sep;26(9):533-9. doi: 10.1038/jhh.2011.67. Epub 2011 Jul 7.

Chapter 13

1. Haze S, Sakai K, Gozu Y. Effects of fragrance inhalation on sympathetic activity in normal adults. Jpn J Pharmacol. 2002;90(3):247-253.

2. Jung DJ et al, "Effects of Ylang-Ylang aroma on blood pressure and heart rate in healthy men", J Exerc Rehabil. 2013 Apr;9(2):250-5. doi: 10.12965/jer.130007. Epub 2013 Apr 25.

3. Russel Hill and Robert Barton, "Psychology: red enhances human performance in contests", Nature. 2005 May 19;435(7040):293.

4. Judge and Cable, "When It Comes to Pay, Do the Thin Win? The Effect of Weight on Pay for Men and Women", Journal of applied psychology, American Psychological Association 2010, Vol. No. 0021-9010/10/

5. http://www.med-grenzfragen.eu/html/geopathy.htm. This site details some of the most up to date information on research in geopathic stress.

6. http://www.medgrenzfragen.eu/download/Geopathy-Gerhard-Hacker-Lithuania08.pdf

7. The Bio-initiative report 2012 . See http://www.bioinitiative.org/

Photography Credits:

Cover Images source www.fotolia.com

Introductory chapter images supplied by www.fotolia.com

Exercise photography supplied by John McDonald https://www.facebook.com/JohnMcDPhotography

All Clip Art supplied by: www.physigraphe.com

About the Author: Clare Rooney

Nationally ranked Athlete

I have been a competitive athlete my whole life and I still continue to train to this day. During my school years I excelled at gymnastics. At university level I made the transition from gymnastics to springboard diving. I trained up to 4 hours daily and won several gold medals at inter-provincial level and national level. When I left Ireland in 1993 to pursue a career in Germany as a Physical Education and Chemistry teacher I got really into the body building culture and spent the next ten years learning everything I could about weight training.

On returning to Ireland and while undertaking multiple internships on strength and conditioning I learned about Olympic lifting. It was while taking an internship in the Eliko training centre in Sweden that the Olympic lifting bug bit. I returned to Ireland and started to train and apply what I had learned. 6 weeks later I had broken all of the national records in my weight division!

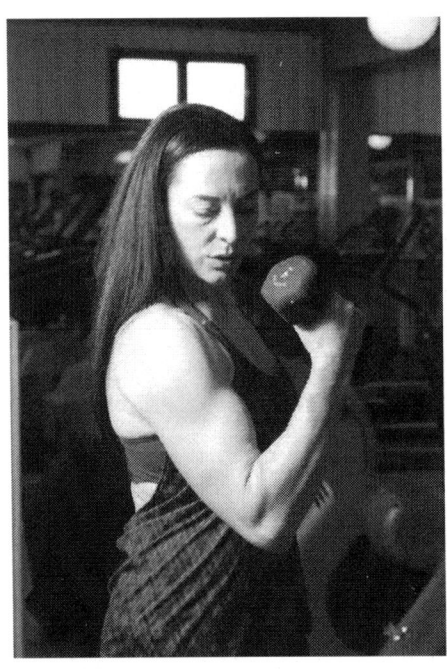

Educational background:

I graduated from the University of Limerick in 1991 with a degree in Physical Education and Chemistry. I worked in Ireland for a brief 2 year stint before heading to Germany where I would remain for 10 years, teaching at the European school in Karlsruhe. It was during my time in Germany that I became exposed to Pilates while visiting a fitness expo. I was so impressed by my initial introduction that I immediately signed up for training. Over the next couple of years and several trips to Cologne later I had trained in mat work and studio apparatus.

It was also during this time that I gained my foundation training as a personal trainer.

On returning to Ireland I set up my personal training business and learned very quickly that the average client had many biomechanical impairments that made standard training highly inappropriate and potentially dangerous.

It was during an expo in the UK that I first heard Paul Chek speak and his message was the same as the lesson I had quickly learned during those early months as a trainer. The average trainee (that's 95 %!) has musculoskeletal issues and imbalances that need to be addressed and corrected first before a conventional weightlifting program can be safely begun. I studied with Paul for several years making frequent trips to California where he has an institute, to Denmark and Sweden and also to the UK. I completed 7 separate internships and truly learned the value of holistic health and how to implement it for my clients.

In the early 90s in Germany I was very into the bodybuilding culture. Anybody who knows anything about the iron game knows the name Charles Poliquin. I knew from reading his articles that this guy was light years ahead of everybody else in his knowledge of how to get the body strong and how to use the modality of training with weights to best effect. I then began training and learning with Charles doing any and all of the internships I could. I repeated some several times to get as much information as I could.

In 1996 I had my first exposure to energy healing while travelling around Mexico. Over the last 19 years I have completed several trainings in diverse method of hands on healing. I have studied copiously about the body's energy field; I have made connections between the science of Quantum Physics and looking at the human body as an energetic entity. I have developed a system of working with the body's energy field using Pilates exercise to balance the body energetically. I have presented at international Pilates conventions and seminars in Germany and Italy on these topics.

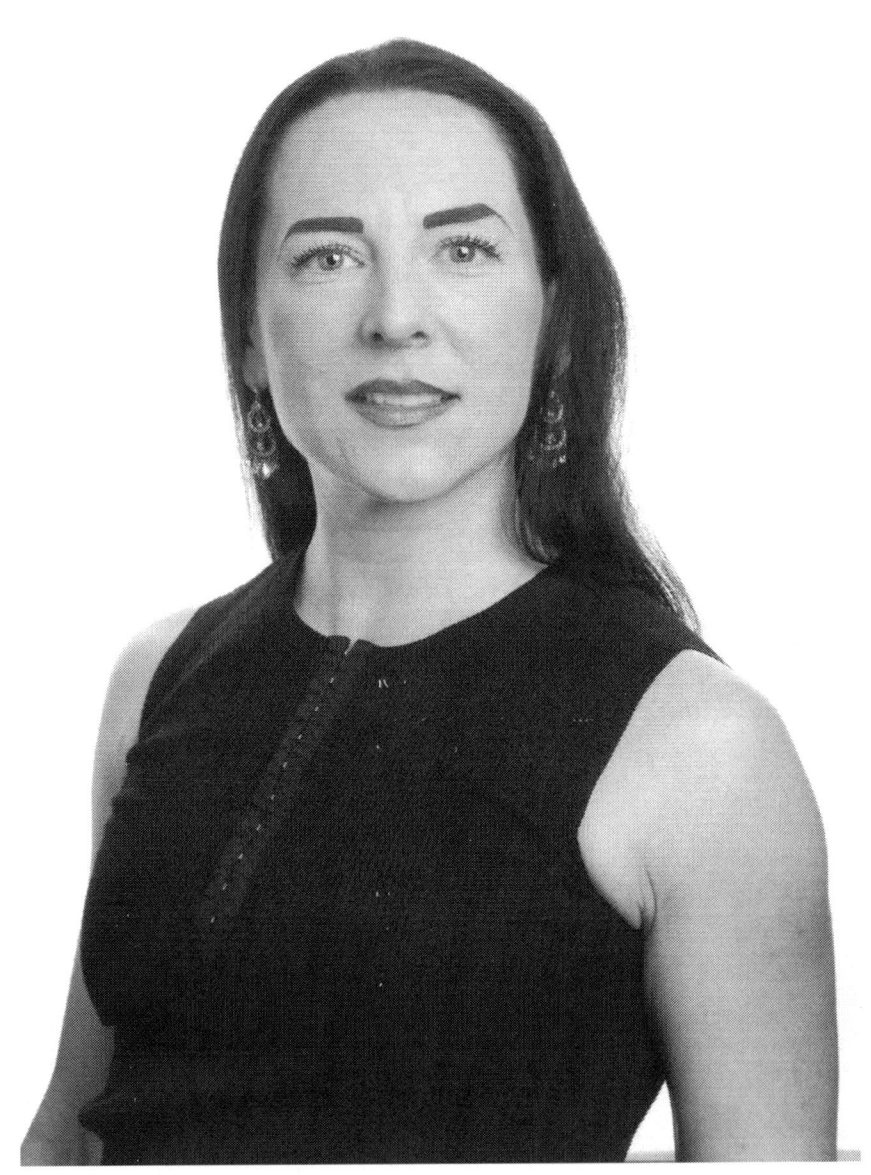

Today I continue to study and travel the world to learn from world leaders in the fields of exercise, functional medicine, nutrition, healing and consciousness.

My Personal Health Challenge

In 1996 I had to give up work for 1 year due to chronic fatigue and severe issues with my spinal alignment. I built myself back up from ground zero (not being able to walk a few hundred metres without being tired) to breaking all of the national records in Olympic lifting. My health challenges which included severe adrenal fatigue , heavy metal poisoning and musculoskeletal breakdown lead me to explore and learn from world experts the real reason I was so unwell. I had to take my whole life apart and eliminate every single stressor . Today I have a vast array of technical knowledge and first hand experience in building health. My biggest message to the public is " its not one thing …its everything". Multiple factors contribute to health and you must learn as many of them as possible to survive in our polluted , stressed and hectic modern world.

It brings me great joy to empower each person I work with to take their health in their own hands. The only person who can heal you is you. You are the creator source of your life, living, reality, body and health. With appropriate tools, awareness and commitment to take action, nothing can stop you from creating the body, the health and the life of your dreams.

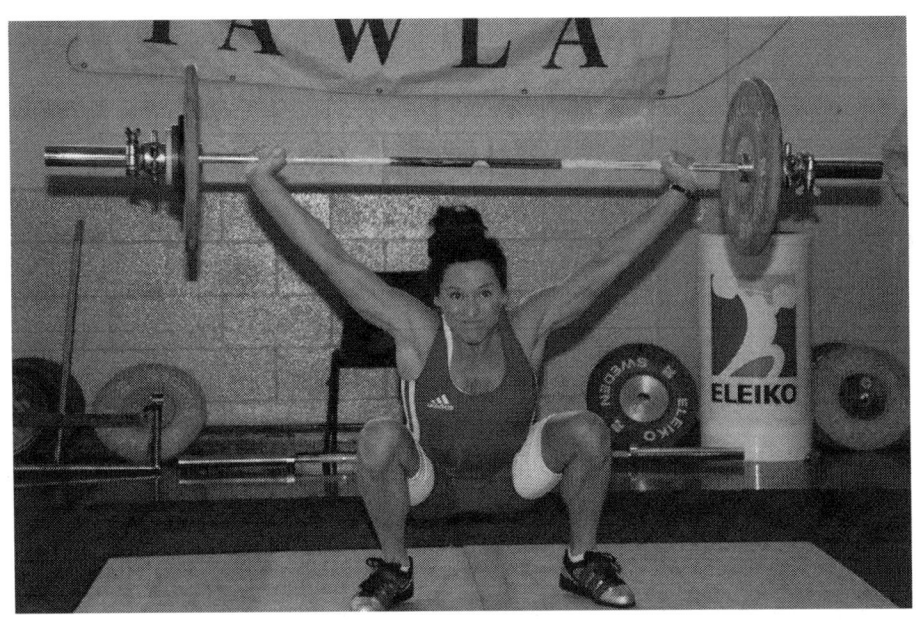

Contact Details:

www.clarerooney.com

info@clarerooney.com

I work with international clients via skype. I offer a range of courses in Nutrition and Lifestyle Coaching which includes assessment of your metabolic type.

Beginners online Pilates course available here:

http://www.clarerooney.com/online-classes/

Made in the USA
Charleston, SC
27 January 2016